RAISING
SAVVY
KIDS

RAISING SAVVY KIDS

TOOLS TO EMPOWER YOUR CHILD TOWARD SUCCESS

ROBIN ANN BURNHAM

Disclaimer

The information provided within this book is for general informational and educational purposes only. The author makes no representations or warranties, express or implied, about the completeness, accuracy, reliability, suitability or availability with respect to the information, products, services, or related graphics contained in this book for any purpose. Any use of this information is at your own risk. This book is not intended as a substitute for the medical advice of physicians. The reader should regularly consult a physician in matters relating to his/her health and particularly with respect to any symptoms that may require diagnosis or medical attention.

Paperback 978-1-7332269-1-2
E-book 978-1-7332269-0-5

DEDICATION

I dedicate this book to my son Brian, for he is the reason I learned the importance of maneuvering life. Suddenly, I was responsible for another. My new role was parent, protector, financier, planner, educator, strategizer and split-second decision maker. He gave me strength, motivation and unconditional love, which has made it all worth the ride.

I also dedicate this book to my Mom and Dad, for they are the reason I am here today. Looking to the future with their guidance, I have evaluated everything I was taught and believed in. I would like to say "Thank You" for they built my foundation that is strong and untouchable. Honesty, trust, integrity, respect, compassion, empathy, and soooo much more.

TABLE OF CONTENTS

INTRODUCTION

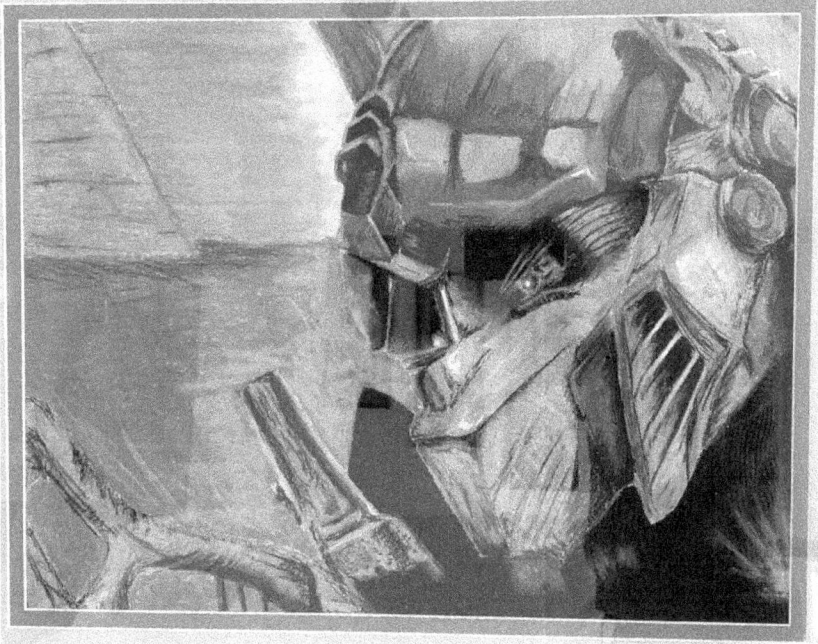

Artist Alisa Chmielinski

STOP! YOU ARE A WARRIOR and your foundation of humanity is under siege. Are you ready to maneuver the battle of life?

- Do you have stone-cold, split-second decision-making ability when life throws you a curveball?

- Is your foundation of ethics, values, and morals cemented in place?

- Do you feel the power of maintaining control and balance in all areas of your life? (The Circle of Wellness) Financial, Physical, Social, Intellectual, Occupational, Environmental, Spiritual, Emotional?

- One step ahead keeps your opponents off guard!

Prepare for your front-line position. This book sets you up to take the WIN. You will be provided with the tools that lead you to become a savvy kid. A kid that successfully maneuvers life and knows what might happen, better yet, what to do when it does! When desire to reach power and balance summons, take one step forward and the gates to success will open, for you will grab the tools.

1. Learn how to build the fortress, keep your foundation strong, and stay within the Circle of Wellness.

2. Answers to potential life emergencies before they happen.

3. A vision of real-life warriors and the careers they have chosen to maneuver in life.

4. A list of industry leaders who provide a clear-cut vision for the future.

This book is your well-thought-out plan, the plan of attack. Arming you with the tools needed to protect and serve, keeping order in the house. Making the right decisions the first time spells success. I promise you, you are important, you are a warrior.

So you ask, "Why should I believe you?" My honest answer to you would be, "I have been there, I have lived it." The initial focus was on my schooling, career, apartment, car, relationship and the challenge of organization and balance. Life changed quickly with new beginnings of marriage, career and the promise of family. The joy of becoming a parent gave me strength, and the devastation of divorce brought me to my knees.

As a single mom with an eight-month-old, it was up to me to make the right decisions without hesitation, for the life of another was now counting on me to do the right thing. A tough battle for one. Backup was summoned, and the goal was to win.

As a parent, it is my responsibility to raise a savvy kid, so when he faces making his own decisions, he can draw from his strength, intellect, instinct, and beliefs. His path became one of success, proven by his character and integrity. We all need support to build strength and be strong. I have living proof that this book provides strength and direction. His name is Brian, he is my son. Brian is intelligent, kind, generous, and he has always had the back of the underdog. He is about building others up, taking charge, and maintaining control in every aspect of his life. He maintains lifelong friendships and accepts others for who they are. His strength is communication and the skill of listening is what propels him to be a leader. I raised Brian by the book. He is the Golden Heart Warrior.

We are living in tumultuous times now. Plan and strategize like a warrior, stay one step ahead of your opponent. Life is a battle, and smooth maneuvering will give you the power and control over your career-finances-family-health-love-happiness and life. This book is your survival guide, your foundation. You will win the war.

CHAPTER 1

THE UNTOUCHABLE FOUNDATION OF INNER STRENGTH

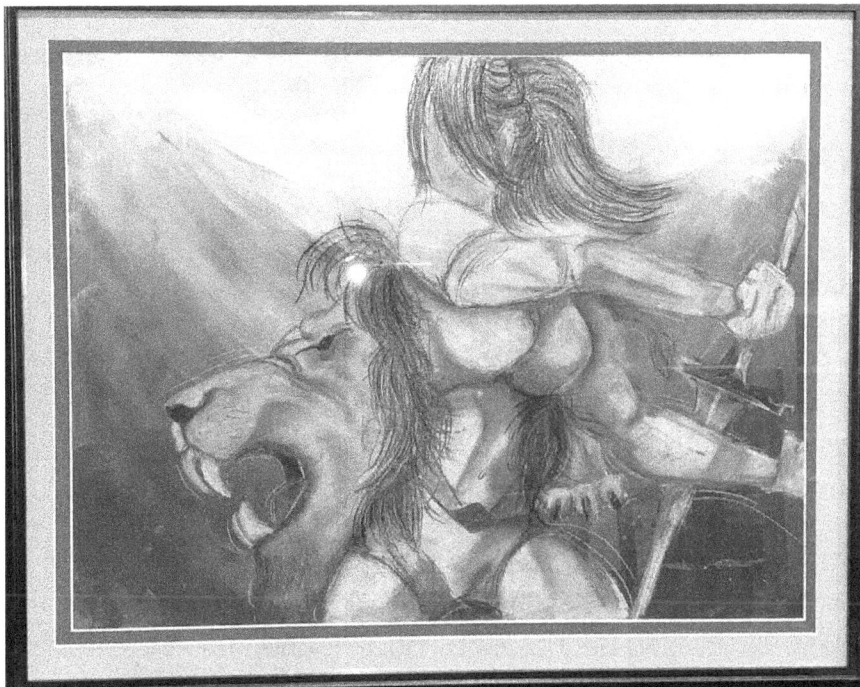

Artist Alisa Chmielinski

Beware! The enemy is lurking. Evil is widespread and stepping slowly toward you. The Warrior must never let his guard down, he must always stay one step ahead. Evil thinks he has won the battle, but you the warrior will win the war!

Evil has no boundaries, shows no mercy, and has no compassion. Lacking foundation—no values, morals, nor sense of decency, it now rears its ugly head. Fear the greed, lies, and false sense of security, it is all in the name of self promotion.

Let your instincts "KICK IN." Sense the smell of deceit, the vision of darkness, and the sound of deafening tones.

Unfortunately for evil, good will triumph. The master plan is to maintain control in all areas of your life, excel as the creator you are, protect your house, and when stable, pay the support forward. Repeat. Repeat. Repeat.

Pull from deep within, rise to the occasion, and build your foundation known as the indestructible fortress. Plug the holes so there can be no infiltration into your world of morals, values, and ethics. You are untouchable and no one can sway you.

We face together the perils of life. Understanding psyche and behavior allows you to read and know instinctively what the next move should be, derailing your opponent's plan to attack.

The actions of evil can, at any moment, fall upon you. The degree of its existence, mild to severe, may be forgiven, but never forgotten. Anger, revenge, hatred, or psychological trauma will present themselves during your lifetime, and a feeling of danger will ensue but will never take you down.

Purposeful, physical attacks known as imminent danger may come with a grave severity. A human being with no conscience may be profiled as a sociopath.

From the world of gangs, ISIS, cults, traffickers, abusers, drugs, or simply killers, let it be known that you may someday have to make a split-second decision to avert a crisis situation.

You see it now, the vision, the path, the importance of becoming strong and savvy. Read on, for you have the key and others are following.

MORALS, VALUES, ETHICS

So they ask, "Who are you?" and "What are you made of?" So what might your response be? You take a strong stance and, unexpectedly, the words begin to flow with ease. You very proudly state your name and the process of building your foundation begins.

Ethics define concepts such as:

> Good vs. Evil
> Right vs. Wrong
> Justice vs. Crime

Your morals are strong because your parents or guardian taught you right from wrong, all the while learning from those who surround you. Learned behaviors shape us into the person we will become. You start to believe, in a certain way, how the world works. You begin to develop a norm of acceptable and unacceptable behavior, and this governs your decision-making. Real-life moral dilemmas pop up regularly in life and you will be asking "What is the right thing to do?" You may just have to trust your experience and conscience.

Question: If you are drinking alcohol at a party, will you drive home?

What will your answer be?

The Ethics Centre provides a non-judgmental forum for the promotion and exploration of ethics and ethical decision-making. One of the Centre's most notable services is its Ethics Counselling Service, free to anyone who may be facing an ethical dilemma. It is believed to be the only service of its kind in the world[1].

A special thank you to Sydney's Ethics Centre for encouraging us to ask ourselves six questions prior to making a decision:

1. Would I be happy if this decision was a headline in the news tomorrow?
2. Is there a rule that applies here?
3. Will the course of action bring a good result?
4. What would happen if everybody did this?
5. What will the course of action do to my character?
6. Is the course of action consistent with the values and principles I believe in and live my life by?

The bottom line about ethics is:

- Who you are and what you stand for
- Development of a well-informed conscience
- Relationships
- Having the courage to explore difficult questions
- Accepting the cost of doing what you think is right
- Asking, What should I do?[2]

The guiding force that points you in the right direction, or what you value to be of the utmost importance and priority is how you will live your life. Personal values are a central part of who you are and who you want to be.

Values evolve as you grow, mature, and gain life experiences. Anyone can influence our values but your life experiences may be one of your strongest teachers.

Value-based decision-making not only shows your sense of right and wrong but also shows integrity. In the end, what's important is your future happiness and satisfaction[3]

"We derive a sense of fulfillment when living our personal values because our motivations and actions are aligned with the aspirations of who we want to be"

~Decision Innovation

I challenge you to determine your top 10 values and then prioritize, for this is who you are. Just a few questions for thought:

- Do your values make you feel good about yourself?
- Would you be proud to tell people you respect and admire what your values are?
- Are your values consistent with your vision for the future?
- Do your values define who you are and want to be?
- Do your values reflect your priorities in life?
- Do your values uplift and motivate you?
- Do your values emphasize your strengths and compensate for your weaknesses?
- Do your values help you in your decision-making?
- Do your values help you in your relationships?
- Are you living a life of meaning?[3] [4]

Are your values consistent with some of the most commonly known values listed below?

- Love
- Peace
- Respect
- Empathy
- Happiness

- Achievement
- Freedom
- Wisdom
- Integrity
- Honesty
- Unconditional love and kindness
- Hard work
- Cooperation
- Compassion
- Forgiveness

Building on ethical values as an executive, or being the leader of your life, comes down to having the same foundation:

- **Honesty**, nothing but the truth
- **Integrity**, even under great pressure, fight for your beliefs
- **Promises**, keep them
- **Loyalty**, avoid undue influences
- **Fairness**, not taking advantage
- **Caring**, help those in need
- **Respect**, respect human dignity regardless of sex, race, or nationality
- **Follow the law**, rules, and regulations
- **Leadership**, taking responsibility and making ethical decisions
- **Accountability**, acknowledge and accept your ethical decisions or lack thereof[5]

The heart of ethics is the integrity and values you behold. They are morals in action with fairness to all. Ethics arm you with the ability to make proper decisions, helping you do the right thing. Morals, values and ethics become the trio that cements your foundation, your Code of Honor.

EMOTIONAL INTELLIGENCE

Your inner strength is building and the feeling that you can not be defeated is growing. When faced with the unknown, it is you who will set aside the reaction and respond with a calmness and authenticity, the making of a leader in control.

"In times of change and uncertainty, having the ability to tap into one's own emotional intelligence becomes crucial. It allows us to connect and understand others on a deeper level".

~Institute for Integrative Nutrition

Ask yourself:

- How quickly do I shift to a positive state after something challenging has happened to me?
- Do I relate to people on a deeper level or do I keep things on the surface?
- Do I tune in to how someone feels during our conversation?[6]

What's in it for me, you ask?

- It will help you stay calm and positive in the face of adversity.
- It keeps relationships healthy, ask yourself three questions:
  Does this need to be said?
  Does this need to be said now?
  Does this need to be said now by me? (Barbiso, Justin 2018 video)
- Improves bonding with others
- Improves decision-making

- Improves self-esteem
- Higher life expectancy
- Motivates to live an authentic lifestyle for peace of mind

"The link between EQ and earnings is so direct that every point increase in EQ adds $1,300 to an annual salary".

-Emotional Intelligence 2.0

Curious About Your Own Emotional Intelligence? Take The Quiz And Find Your Healthy Sense Of Self (www.healthysenseofself.com/emotional-intelligence)[7]

Rising to the level of success continues, you are becoming a force to be reckoned with.

Feel your feelings, know what they mean and how they affect others.

- Know your strengths and weaknesses and choose how you react.
- Stay in control, do not compromise values, admit your mistakes, and stay calm.
- Work your goals, find one positive aspect of a challenging situation.
- Show you care.
- Negotiate and compromise—with respect and patience[6].

What signs do you possess? **Check below:**

- ❑ Do you stop and think before you speak?
- ❑ Is your response to emotions controlled, or do you react?

- ❑ Can you look to criticism as an opportunity to learn? Can it make you better?
- ❑ Are you authentic?
- ❑ Do you say what you mean and mean what you say?
- ❑ Do you stick to your values and principles?
- ❑ Can you put yourself in someone else's shoes to be empathetic to their situation and stop judging?
- ❑ Do you acknowledge and appreciate others?
- ❑ Do you inspire others to be their best to build trust?
- ❑ Do you give constructive criticism so others see it as helpful?
- ❑ Do you have the strength and courage to apologize, even if you're not wrong, showing value to the relationship?
- ❑ Can you forgive and forget, allowing yourself to move forward?
- ❑ Do you keep your commitments showing reliability and trustworthiness?
- ❑ Do you help others? It will build trust.
- ❑ Are you ready to protect yourself from others' manipulations by keeping your emotional intelligence sharp?[8]

KEEP IN MIND

Mind control is known as manipulation, thought reform, brainwashing, mental control, and coercive persuasion. An attempt to influence and persuade others to change their beliefs and behaviors for someone else's benefit. This can lead to a significant disruption to an individual at their very core. The deepest level of their identity such as values, beliefs, decisions, behaviors, or relationships.

It is a subtle process, meaning you will not be aware of the extent of influence being imposed on you. You will believe that you are the decision maker but it is not so.

Coercion can change behavior, but coercive persuasion (mind control) will change attitude and behavior.

Watch out for the tricksters for they will try to take you to the darkside, but now you know. Beware of the socio-paths, psychopaths and manipulators who have no conscience. Everyone is susceptible and that means you.

Your protection is understanding the workings and tactics used to control and recruit[9].

If subjected to mind control in any form and to any degree, your internal warning will sound, the red flags will rise. Listen and trust your instincts for they will protect you. For those that are vulnerable and may fall prey, the path will self-correct if it is allowed to assist. Warning received, now believe you are smarter than the enemy.

Take charge, maintain control, and no one can break you. The ultimate strength will never allow another to alter your thoughts or your sense of direction. Keep in mind:

The way you think is the way you go, if you are handed lemons make lemonade, and for the view on life, do you see a half-glass of water as half full or empty?

THE CONFLICT CURE

Human conflict needs no invitation and the two of you will meet up sooner than later. The Savvy Kid is prepared for what is to come and will handle the matter despite its intensity.

The puzzle to resolving conflict. How many pieces do you possess? **Check below:**

- ❏ Accept the conflict as a natural unavoidable occurrence
- ❏ Remain calm to avoid escalation
- ❏ Listen carefully and work through how you feel
- ❏ Analyze why it happened and how it can be resolved
- ❏ Use neutral language by avoiding inflammatory words
- ❏ Separate the person from the problem
- ❏ Work together
- ❏ Agree to disagree
- ❏ Focus on the future
- ❏ Move past your position and compromise
- ❏ Share interests
- ❏ Keep confidentiality[10]

LEADERS LOVE CONTROL

You, the controller, dictator, creator, and architect, decide the next plan of attack. The path you see fit, now forge on and prove yourself. You control your own destiny. The golden rule is "Keep your friends close and your enemies closer."

- Are you a high performer?
- Can you manage your own life?
- Are you confident?
- Are you optimistic?
- Are you open to change?
- Are you decisive?[11]

Lead your life effectively using four basic fundamentals:

1. Know your strengths and weaknesses.

   You are truly strong when you have the ability to influence others' actions, decisions, and opinions in a positive way that will benefit and empower others. Tapping into one's intellect, connecting with their well-being and working together will set an example of caring and set an example of leadership.

Do you possess the qualities of a leader? **Check below:**

- ❑ Honesty
- ❑ Integrity
- ❑ Trust
- ❑ Self-control
- ❑ Confident
- ❑ Boldness
- ❑ Value directness
- ❑ Balance honesty with care and compassion

Do you possess qualities of a strong leader?

- ❑ Self-Control or Impulsiveness?
- ❑ Tenacity or Laziness?
- ❑ Boldness or Hesitancy?
- ❑ Honesty or Deceitfulness?
- ❑ Focus on results or Aimlessness?
- ❑ Confidence or Insecurity?
- ❑ Pragmatism or Impracticality?
- ❑ Decisiveness or Indecisiveness?

2. Write and speak clearly, use active listening.

   Be attentive and recap conversations to show understanding.

3. Communicate your vision, align the efforts of others and build commitment.

4. Learn, value, and seek experiences.

Building leadership skills the natural way brings results. You may hear these tips often from friends, family, and mentors. Learn from your mistakes, ask insightful questions and be open to feedback. This advice could come in handy in a big way[12].

inspiration

Head, Heart and Gut
Lodestars of Powerful Decision Making
by Lee Milteer

We are living in unprecedented times of stress, confusion and overwhelm. We all need resources to help navigate these challenging times and make the right decisions for the highest and best long-term good for ourselves, our families and our businesses.

Those resources can be found within each of us if we pause to consider three reliable indicators: the head (intellect), the heart (feelings) and the gut (intuition). Before proceeding in making an important choice, make a habit of checking these built-in sensors, which can warn us about

danger or give us the go-ahead.

Head: Make use of intellect and past knowledge. All decisions, actions and even non-actions have repercussions. Use the conscious mind to discern questions that need to be answered. For example, is this person telling the truth? What has worked in the past? Have we done our due diligence and homework before making a decision?

Heart: I listen to my heart and ask: Is this the right direction for me? Do I naturally feel attracted to this? Am I hearing truth?

The internal part of us, the voice inside, tells us when things feel right or wrong. For example, are we relaxed around the person we are asking the question about, or do we feel uptight and uncomfortable? Keep in mind that our bodies do talk to us. For me personally, if I feel shut down, tight and not good, I know something is not right. However, if I feel open, lighthearted and relaxed, I trust that my heart is telling me that, "All is well." We have to pay attention to our own internal signals.

Gut: We need to trust our intuition. If it doesn't feel right, chances are it's not right for us. What may be right for one person can be wrong for another. Our gut instinct, our inner voice, is always there for us when we take the time to pay attention and listen. Become conscious, and do not go into the default mode of past decisions or behaviors. Life has changed and requires more awareness of what is truth and what is not, and we need to utilize our senses, not the old programmed beliefs from others. It is our job to use the instincts that we have to help navigate new terrain.

Lee Milteer is the author of Reclaim the Magic: The Real Secrets to Manifesting Anything You Want *and an award-winning speaker and life and business strategist. Sign up for her free weekly Gems of Wisdom newsletter at Milteer.com. Go to FiveTypesOfEnergy.com for a free copy of her "Five Types of Energy" video series.*

Milteer, Lee. (2019) Head, Heart and Gut. Albany, New York: Albanyhappenings.com[13]

INTUITION YOUR SIXTH SENSE

A Warrior knows when the enemy is approaching before they appear, as he looks into the distance, a feeling of uneasiness occurs, the time has come.

A view of intuition is like the north star of the human soul, an inner guide that helps us navigate the different landscapes of life. True intuition arises from within the depths of your soul. It speaks in the language of spirit - love, flow, hope, and forward movement. Similar but different is instinct, the physiological language - survival, fight or flight, judgement, avoidance, aggression, and fear. An internal gift presents itself, and if you heed the call, grace will lift you like the invisible upwind just as you step out over the unknown and it will carry you to the place where you need to be. A giant leap in your development, awareness, and understanding[14].

Instincts are to be trusted, they will protect you, and someday may save your life. It is time to listen quietly and heed the advice.

"In the year 2014, The Office of Naval Research embarked on a four-year $3.85 million dollar program to explore the phenomena of premonition and intuition. The Pentagon's focus was to maximize the power of the sixth sense for operational use. The power of intuition helped our troops to make quick judgments during combat that ended up saving lives"[15].

Intuition is the one ability you are born with. Your guiding "inner voice" which always knows the truth - what is ultimately best for you, in all situations. Your dreams, mental imagery, vibes, coincidences, insights, and gut feelings may be trying to tell you something. Meditation is the best tool to access your subconscious, and awaken your super-powerful, yet dormant intuition. Dig through the noise, mental chatter, anxiety, self interest, body tension, emotional push-pull, and material world attachment, to the magnificence of your subconscious mind[16].

Wisdom of the successful:

- Listen to your inner voice
- Take time for solitude
- Be creative
- Practice meditation and mindfulness

- Observe your surroundings and notice when odd things happen
- Listen to your body particularly those gut feelings.
- Connect deeply with others
- Pay attention to your dreams
- Enjoy plenty of downtime
- Let go of negative emotions[17]

Intuition speaks in many forms, are you listening?:

Sometimes, it is that peaceful feeling in your heart, a tightness in your chest or that sinking feeling in your gut.
You will feel confidence and clarity when it speaks.
You may notice the same opportunities keep knocking at your door.
You find clarity when you take your mind off what you are seeking. One of those "ah-ha!" moments.
You may notice your thoughts are being pulled in a certain direction. The thoughts that seem to "pop" in out of nowhere.
A particular thought keeps popping up in your head. The thought just will not go away.
You will feel inspired and excited.
The more you listen, the happier and secure you may feel about the choices you make[18].

"You are what you expect when you trust yourself, you tend to prove yourself right. When you believe in the availability of your own answers, they tend to show up at the right time. It is a psychological primer for future performance."[19]

~Scott Ginsberg

How Intuitive Are You? Take The Quiz And Know Your 6th Sense Score https://www.finerminds.com/mind-power/how-intuitive-are-you-quiz/[20].

EMPATHY AND SYMPATHY

This topic pulls at your heartstrings, something that we all will face in our lifetime. That moment when you find yourself going to the store to buy a sympathy card. Something has happened to someone you know and they have left someone behind. You understand the person left behind will be grieving and sadness has set in. Sympathy is called the "I'm sorry compassion" because you understand how they are feeling. These things we wish were not so, but you will not escape this one, so be prepared.

Have you ever heard the saying "Do not judge a book by its cover?" Sometimes things are not what they appear to be. Or maybe you have heard "Do not judge someone until you have walked a mile in their shoes." They call this empathy, because with great sincerity, you try to understand what the other person is going through. Envision what it would feel like if you were them, and what they were going through, that it was happening to you.

The time has come when you are face to face with the suffering of another. Physical, mental, or emotional suffering does not discriminate. You now experience the push or pull to act, the motivation to help alleviate or prevent it. Compassion is its name and it is that we are all thankful for. The smallest act of compassion can have the biggest impact.

"The simple act of listening with your full presence can be one of the most compassionate acts you can offer"[21].

~ Sara Schairer

Which qualities of compassion do you possess?. **Check below:**

- ❑ Patience
- ❑ Wisdom
- ❑ Kindness
- ❑ Perseverance
- ❑ Warmth
- ❑ Resolve[22]

Believe in and allow yourself to:

- Listen and offer the gift of your presence
- Hold off on the advice
- Allow others to be emotional
- Ask questions
- Be authentic

How empathetic are you? Check your empathy score at: https://greatergood.berkeley.edu/quizzes/take_quiz/empathy[23]

WAREMPATH

Do you have the gift of observation, connection, sensitivity to others' emotions, and energies? Are you bold, courageous, fearless, and strong? If so, you are an empath warrior. You know you are called to do something greater.

The four signs of the empath warrior:

1. You daydream often.
2. You have big visions.
3. You depend on encouragement.
4. You struggle with self-care, you see it as being selfish[24].

The warrior spirit stays strong and thrives by taking advantage of strategic, energy-saving tools:

- Expressing gratitude
- Meditation
- Mindful breathing
- Strengthened intuition
- Loving yourself[25]

It is okay to be vulnerable and strong at the same time. Go forward and develop your compassion, intuition, depth, and a deep connection with others.

HABITS AT THE HIGHEST LEVEL

The Savvy Kid and Warrior are skillful and mindful for they are one. They envision what will be and how to get there through sheer determination, a mindset that is unswayable and impenetrable.

Building power and control with routine discipline shows balance, the wellness that is deserving of success.

Have you known someone who had it all and lost it because their inner foundation was weak?

Loss of family due to cheating?
Loss of job due to stealing or most recently in the news for harassment?
Loss of everything, including life due to addiction?

This will not be in your vision for your inner foundation refuses to allow negative forces to intervene. You will rise above and pull others to safety, you are aware and prepared for the worst. Your maneuvering will be calculated and smooth. Others will follow in your footsteps. . .

The strength of the mind now sets the stage. Stephen Covey's *7 Habits of Highly Effective People* speaks of powerful lessons for personal change. Thank you to Fearless Motivation for revealing quotes by Stephen Covey:

"Make time for planning: Wars are won in
the general's tent."

~Stephen Covey

"A personal mission statement becomes the DNA for
every other decision we make."

~Stephen Covey

"Every human has four endowments - self-awareness,
conscience, independent will and creative
imagination. These give us the ultimate human
freedom. The power to choose, to respond,
to change."[26]

~Stephen Covey

How many habits do you possess or seek to change, for only the strong survive? **Check below:**

- ❏ Be Proactive, take initiative, and make things happen. You are the creator of your life and only you choose your response to any given situation. Freedom is power to achieve growth and happiness.
- ❏ Begin with the end in mind, you can create the future in your mind, imagine it, see it. Envision, see the potential, create in your mind what we cannot at the present time see with our eyes.
- ❏ Put first things first, focus on the important things in life. Willpower and creating a clear-cut understanding of what needs to be will get you where you want to go.
- ❏ Think "Win-Win"—it produces profit, power, recognition for everybody.
- ❏ Seek first to Understand, then to be Understood—listening to understand requires respect and restraint.
- ❏ Synergize. Build teamwork, unity, and creativity
- ❏ Sharpen the Saw. Renewal is the most important thing—you continually improve, innovate, and refine[27].

Chapter 2

FINANCIAL FUNDING AND THE COST OF STRATEGY

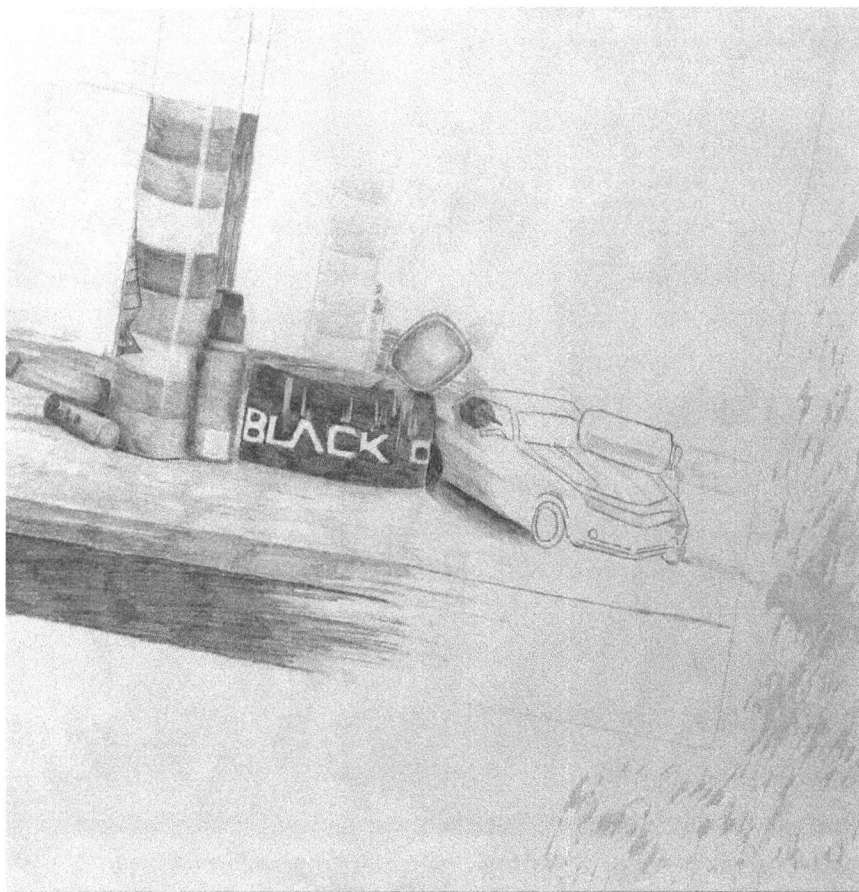

Artist Alisa Chmielinski

The foundation is laid and it is time to forge to the next level, strengthening the plan and maintaining control weakens the opponent.

The inner financial workings could make or break you. The warrior has shown the strength to build, the mind control to strategize, and now prepares to move forward. The thought is to always stay one step ahead, and be ready to abort any crisis that should arise, keeping the path to the win clear. It would be a costly mistake to underestimate the need for funding. From this day forward, money is of no object. For the emotions run high and the budget has been set. The battle must begin.

COST-OF-LIVING EXPENSES

Financial Control. "Cash is King," only the truth lies within success. The greedy may obtain short-term success, but it is not sustainable, eventually it takes it toll and the wiser see through the con. The ultimate goal is to obtain financial stability, then begin helping others. Some speak the truth of giving when suddenly positive happenings begin to blossom. It has been mentioned that in our three levels of financial class—low/middle/high, our middle class may be at risk. If so, will you go high or low? Beware, your opponent will try to break you, it is of the utmost importance to stay in the game and on your game! What will your next move be?

FINANCIAL FREEDOM

Financial freedom has a sophisticated ring to it. The goal is to be able to make stress-free, money-making decisions, decreasing the burden of money concerns.

Manage your money and budget monthly, base it on your income, not your debt, and save whenever possible. What will help you? **Check below:**

- ❏ Make a grocery list
- ❏ Download coupon apps
- ❏ Shop at a dollar store
- ❏ Cook dinner at home
- ❏ Set up bill reminders
- ❏ Money saving purchases (reusable water bottle/light bulbs/programmable thermostat)
- ❏ Pay off debt, starting with the smallest to the largest bill (minimum payment on all but the smallest bill)
- ❏ Cut up your credit cards and ask the card company to lower your interest rate
- ❏ Never carry a car payment
- ❏ Rent vs buying a home
- ❏ Wanted and desired items shall wait until you meet financial freedom personally
- ❏ Make extra payments
- ❏ Transfer a high-interest balance to a credit card with zero % APR
- ❏ Check unclaimed money at MissingMoney.com and Unclaimed.org
- ❏ Check HUD.gov for unknown Refund Money (FHA loan)
- ❏ Refinance student loan debt
- ❏ Reduce utility bills
- ❏ Find cheaper car insurance
- ❏ Coupons and Groupon for lower rates
- ❏ Check bank statements daily for fraudulent charges
- ❏ Get a cheaper cell phone service
- ❏ Eliminate fees (Investment/ATM/Checking)
- ❏ Ask your credit card company to waive a late fee

❑ Cut Subscriptions[28]

Know your creditworthiness, your credit score is your report card on your financial health. Check your credit reports yearly. Stay sharp because they make mistakes, so check for errors. A bill may be on the report that you didn't know about or you forgot about. Bill collections remain on your report for seven years, even after you pay it off.

AnnualCreditReport.com is free one time a year, any more than this will ding your credit. Monitor your credit for free at Credit Karma[29].

"Building wealth is impossible if you're living paycheck to paycheck. Give every dollar a name before the month begins, and track your spending throughout the month."

~Chris Hogan

Be smart about your career:

- Is there income earning potential with advancement?
- Do you enjoy the work?
- Do the benefits of retirement and healthcare meet your goals?

Strategize Savings:

- Pay yourself first before expenses
- Automate your withdrawals
- Save $1,000 for an emergency fund
- Save three to six months' worth of expenses when stable

- Increase savings starting point at 1% income, increase to 5%/10%/15%/20%/30% for retirement funds
- Savings for big items (vacation)

Investments:

- Start retirement funds and maximize employer matching amounts only (401k/Roth/Traditional IRA)
- Tax-free accounts (employer health care spending (HSA))
- Obtain a financial advisor for guidance
- Invest in yourself (look professional)
- Purchase real estate (pay off home and then purchase a home for rentals)
- Monitor your investments
- 10/10/10 Plan is 10% to investments, 10% to savings, 10% to charity (pay yourself first)[30]

Tips for buying a used car:

Free VIN Report prior to buying a used car which lists any accidents with an insurance claim and registrations by state and type of title:

- Check Free VehicleHistory.com or ISeeCars.com/VIN
- Use CarFax, vehicle inspection, and test drive to make the best decision.

Have a mechanic check the car, it is not against the law for the seller to be dishonest about the condition of the car. Use ASE.com (Automotive Service Excellence) and check for an independent mechanic near you. Look for the Blue Seal Program. Watch out for flood-damaged vehicles and failed electrical systems[31].

Tax Preparation checklists can be found at DaveRamsey.com:

- Tax Prep Checklist (Income/Common Deductions)
- Small Business Tax Prep Checklist (Itemized Business Expense)[32]

FINANCIAL TIPS

Financial advisement has taken a turn for the better. The word is out that the #1 priority is to deal with a Fiduciary.

"In a fiduciary relationship, one person, in a position of vulnerability, justifiably vests confidence, good faith, reliance, and trust in another whose aid, advice, or protection is sought in some matter. In such a relation good conscience requires the fiduciary to act at all times for the sole benefit and interest of the one who trusts."[33]

~Wikipedia

Your financial portfolio should be diversified into different areas or as the saying goes "Don't put all your eggs in the same basket."

So many choices exist - stocks and stock mutual funds, corporate and municipal bonds, bond mutual funds, lifecycle funds, exchange-traded funds, money market funds, and U.S. Treasury securities.

The three most popular asset categories are stocks, bonds, and cash.

Stocks are a portfolios "heavy hitter," offering the greatest potential for growth, but due to the volatile nature, loss can occur.

Bonds are generally less volatile than stocks but offer more modest returns.

Cash and cash equivalents-such as savings deposits, certificates of deposit, treasury bills, money market deposit accounts, and money market funds- are the safest investments but offer the lowest return of the three categories mentioned[34].

FINRA (Financial Industry Regulatory Authority) protects you as an investor, keeping your best interests at heart:

- Anyone who sells securities has been tested, qualified, and licensed.
- Security advertisements are monitored to be truthful and not misleading.
- Securities products sold to investors will be suitable to their needs.
- Investors are given full disclosure about the product before they purchase.
- Deter misconduct by enforcing the rules and discipline for those who break the rules.
- Prevent wrongdoing in the US markets.
- Educates and informs investors.
- The Broker check allows investors to research professionals.
- Offers an Online Fund Analyzer.
- Resolves securities disputes.

Use FINRA.org for free resources and check your Risk/Scam meter. Is your opportunity too good to be true? (https://www.finra.org/)

The Rule of 72 is a simple equation that will help you determine how long an investment will take to double, given a fixed interest rate. This shows the value of why there is a need to start retirement savings early.

Divide 72 by the interest rate and you will get the number of years it will take to double your money:

> Example. $1000 investment 72 / 10% =
> 7.2 years = $2,000
> 14.4 years = $4,000
> 21.6 years = $8,000
> 28.8 years = $16,000

Grab your Rule of 72 cheat sheet now[35]:
https://www.ruleoneinvesting.com/blog/financial-control/using-the-rule-of-72/

THE MONEY BOSS

Financial independence is a process with different stages. More than just a theory. The Money Boss shows "The Road To Financial Freedom," and its six stages in the photo below[36].

MONEY BO$S

MASTER YOUR MONEY – AND YOUR LIFE

THE ROAD TO FINANCIAL FREEDOM

STAGE 0 - DEPENDENCE

Your lifestyle depends on others for financial support. You're in this stage if your parents still give you money. You're in this stage if you spend more than you earn. You're in this stage if your debt payments exceed your income.

STAGE 1 - SOLVENCY

You can meet your financial commitments without outside help. You reach this stage when you begin earning a "profit", when your income exceeds your expenses. You're using the surplus to repay debt and to meet immediate financial obligations.

STAGE 2 - STABILITY

You no longer have consumer debt. You've repaid your credit cards, auto loans, and so on. You may still have some "good debt" – college loans, a mortgage – but you've eliminated other obligations *and* built a buffer of emergency savings to protect yourself from unfortunate events.

STAGE 3 - AGENCY

You have the freedom to live and work as you choose. You've eliminated *all* debt, including student loans and mortgage (or you have the cash to do so, if you wanted). You have enough banked that you could quit your job at a moment's notice and feel no trepidation for the future.

STAGE 4 - SECURITY

Your investment income covers your basic needs. The money you've saved and invested would fund simple housing, basic food, essential clothing, and insurance – even if you never worked another day in your life.

STAGE 5 - INDEPENDENCE

Your investment income supports your current standard of living. The money you've saved and invested would allow you to live like you do today...until the day you die. It covers the basics *and* creature comforts. You have enough.

STAGE 6 - ABUNDANCE

You have enough – and then some. Your passive income from all sources will not only fund your lifestyle forever, but also grant you the freedom to do whatever you choose: indulge in luxury, build a business empire, explore the world.

Visit moneyboss.com to learn more about financial freedom.

80/20 YOUR LIFE

The 80/20 Rule is considered to be one of the most helpful concepts for life and time management. A small effort equals a big reward, 20% effort = 80% results.

Make a list of 10 things that are the most important to accomplish. Now two of the items on your list will be worth more than the other eight added together.

These will most likely be the hardest and most complex of all your goals. Believe in yourself and your work, because the payoff and reward can be tremendous. Put the small things to the side because they are of the lowest value to you.

They say the attitude of the wealthy is to work on one big goal all the time, and if you do, you too can change your life.

"When your goals are clear, you will come up with exactly the right answer at exactly the right time."

~Brian Tracy

The starting point of success and achievement has always been to dream big about the wonderful things that you can become, have, and do.

A wise man once said: "You must dream big dreams, for only big dreams have the power to move the minds of men."

~Brian Tracy

Dreaming big increases self-esteem and self-confidence. You will feel more powerful about yourself and your ability to deal with what happens to you.

Living the 80/20 Rule without limits or constraint requires you to:

- Be clear on who you are, what you want, and where you want to go.
- Write down your goals and make plans to accomplish them by working on them every day.
- Apply the 80/20 to everything you do, focus on becoming outstanding in 20% of your tasks that contribute to 80% percent of your results.
- Learn on a continuous basis.
- Concentration requires self-discipline, so force yourself to focus on one goal until complete[37]

The 80/20 Principle in everyday life increases efficiency:

- What 20% of your time do you spend doing, that gives you 80% happiness?
- What 20% of your clothes do you wear 80% of the time?
- What 20% of healthy food do you eat 80% of the time?
- What 20% of your conversations create 80% intimacy with your partner?
- What 20% of your work gets you 80% credit and recognition?[38]

THE GOLDEN CREDIT REPORT AND CREDIT SCORE

The famous "Credit Report" and yes, you are being watched and tracked. Depending on how you behave, your actions will impact your buying power. If you decide to neglect the bills, then they will succeed in taking you down, and if you pay your bills in a timely manner then you will be rewarded with a great score. When the time comes that you need a loan to purchase a home or something of great importance to you, the score is everything. The credit report is a crucial tool that tells the story of where you stand financially, and will also show signs if someone has stolen your identity. The report includes where you have lived, how you pay your bills, if you have been sued, or filed for bankruptcy. The credit score is a numerical value of the information in your report, scaling between 300 and 850, 300 being the lowest. This calculates the risk you pose to lenders and trickles downhill to employers as well. The question they have formed is "How likely is it that you will pay them back?"

You are eligible to receive one free copy every year from all three reporting credit bureau agencies, Equifax / Transunion / Experian. You will receive the report only, but you will be given the opportunity to pay if you would like to improve the score. Free credit monitoring from Credit Karma will show your credit score, but keep in mind, it is the NON-FICO score[39].

Any employer can request a report on you, check to see what they have on you at:

TheWorkNumber.com or call 1-866-604-6570 per Clark Howard.

If you freeze your reports due to Identity theft, you may receive a Free Report.

Challenge Errors on your Credit Report. Black marks on your report can mean:

- Job denial
- High-interest rates on loans
- High insurance rates
- Denied credit

Your true Credit Score is your FICO Score, and this shows your creditworthiness. Your Credit score may show codes along with it. Go to ReasonCode.org to decipher what the lenders are actually saying about you.

Breakdown of the score calculation includes:

- 35% payment history
- 30% amount owed
- 15% the length of your credit history
- 10% new credit
- 10% mix of credit

Causes for your score to drop:

- Late/missed payments
- Maxed out credit card
- Applying for a new credit card
- No or little credit history

Financial institutions have developed an array of products and services, such as secured credit cards and credit builder loans, tailored to help consumers new to credit who want to establish and build credit. A secured credit card requires a cash deposit and that generally acts as the available balance for the card.

Focus on improving your credit score and maintain good credit:

- Check report and fix errors
- Pay off small debts
- Make multiple payments monthly
- Pay attention to the balances
- Do not charge over 30% of allowable credit
- Pay on time *****PRIORITY*****
- Build credit, get a card, charge a small amount, and pay off immediately
- Do not open a credit card or buy a car right before applying for a mortgage[29] [40]

Dave Ramsey's *7 Baby Steps* program is a step-by-step plan that shows you how to get out of debt and save money. The plan goes beyond simply treating the symptoms of money problems like debt and lack of savings. The plan, Financial Peace University, is a nine-week course on money management. The outline goes like this:

Step 1. Save $1000 for emergency.
Step 2. Pay off debt using snowball method.
Step 3. Save three to six months of expenses for emergencies.
Step 4. Invest 15% of your household income into Roth IRA and pre-tax retirement.
Step 5. Save for your child's college fund.
Step 6. Pay off your home.
Step 7. Build wealth and give back[41].

THREE STYLES OF SUCCESS

"You cannot make progress without making decisions."

~ Jim Rohn

Decision-making is a non-negotiable experience that you will encounter at some point in your life. Prepare for the confrontation, because it is coming your way. Successful people look at the bigger picture and foresee long-term results, they know smart decisions are necessary to thrive, achieve, and sustain success in life.

Warren Buffet utilizes a method that helps him make the right decisions the first time, it is the 10/10/10 Rule. Ask yourself three questions when you need to make a decision:

#1- How will I feel about my decision in 10 minutes?
#2- How will I feel about my decision in 10 months?
#3- How will I feel about my decision in 10 years?

The brain is wired to want short-term pleasure, but looking at the long-term gratifications and ramifications (balance due on your credit card) allows you to make smarter decisions.

Think further ahead, and think smarter, it will save you from a typical immediate reaction. Smart decisions bring you a step closer to financial freedom, happiness, and wealth.

"Avoiding rash decisions comes with practice. Many people who seem in control and constantly avoid them are able to do so because they have been practicing and building that muscle all their life. They go through a constant feedback loop of decision analysis-continuously improving their decision-making capabilities."[42]

~Adam Fortuna (Minafi.com)

Brian Tracy offers a seven-point Formula to keep you on the road to success, keep on believing in yourself:

- Think Positive about money, money is not evil because it helps so many, and money can help with happiness. Have you ever seen a child's face when they receive a gift?
- Write and rewrite your goals.
- Plan your day, and you will become sharper and more precise in all that you do, better focus and a greater sense of control (personal power).
- Concentration is absolutely essential, focus on what will make you the most money.
- Invest in yourself, listen to audio tapes in the car, money management and personal finance are a must.
- Ask yourself two questions after each meeting or event:

#1- What did I do right?

#2- What would I do differently next time?

- Be generous to others, treat them as the most important person in the world.

Money is essential to happiness, and material prosperity predicts life satisfaction.

Financial freedom is the development of specific habits.

Which ones do you possess? **Check below:**

- ❑ Be frugal with every penny and every dollar.
- ❑ Save money, pay yourself first.
- ❑ Overcome obstacles because you do deserve to have financial freedom.
- ❑ Believe in yourself because money opens doors.
- ❑ Recognize and accept that virtually everyone who has money was once broke.
- ❑ Take action and become a student of money[43].

Rich Dad Poor Dad, **Robert Kiyosaki** offers his financial expertise to be creative in making money. Acquire assets to offset the cost of whatever you want to buy, not live below your means.

"The Cashflow Quadrant." Which one do fall into?
Check below:

- ❑ Employee - pays the most taxes and trades time for money
- ❑ Self-Employed or Specialist - pays the most taxes and trades time for money
- ❑ Big Business - pays the least taxes, produces cash flow
- ❑ Investor - pays the least taxes and produces cash flow

Three types of income:

- Earned - money from a paycheck
- Portfolio - money from stocks
- Passive - money that generates money (personal communication from The Rich Dad Company, 5, May, 2018)

WATCH YOUR BACK AND LOOK OVER YOUR SHOULDER

"Watch your back and look over your shoulder," your opponent has been watching every move you make, and they are ready to infiltrate! Are you ready for the battle? They want your identity, cash, and whatever else they can get. Draw a line in the sand and if they cross it, unleash the troops. They will pay the price.

BBB Better Business Bureau says that if you abide by 10 simple recommendations you will avoid most attempts at Scams and Fraud:

1. Never send money to someone you have never met. No wire transfers, gift or prepaid debit cards because they cannot be traced.
2. Do not click on links or open attachments in unsolicited email. Links can download unsolicited email. Links can download malware on your computer and steal your identity.
3. Do not believe everything you see. (They mimic official seals, fonts, and other details, such as caller ID).
4. Do not buy online unless a transaction is secure. Check out the company on BBB.org.
5. Be cautious when dealing with anyone you have met online. (Dating websites, Craigslist, or social media).
6. Never share personal identifiable information if contacted by someone soliciting by phone/email/door.
7. Do not be pressured to act immediately.

8. Use secure, traceable transactions when making payments. Say no to high pressure tactics such as cash payments, cash-only deals, high upfront payments, over-payments, or handshake deals.
9. Work with local businesses. Check them out on BBB.org. They should have proper ID, licensing, and insurance (especially contractors coming into your home).
10. Be cautious about what you share on social media. Use the privacy settings.[44]

Protect yourself against credit card fraud:

- Keep it in a safe place (card, card number, and phone number to call if stolen)
- Keep it to yourself (never relinquish the information unless legit)
- Keep it memorable (passwords and PIN numbers)
- Shred it (all identifiable personal information)
- Take it (never leave receipts behind)
- Sign it (the back of your cards)[45]

It is almost unbelievable that Equifax, the major credit reporting agency that holds all of our personal financial data, was hacked in what is now being called the Equifax Data Breach. Our Social Security numbers, birth dates, addresses, and drivers licenses were accessed. If you were impacted, Equifax offers you a free credit monitoring service with Trustedid.com.

The FTC Federal Trade Commission offers information on how to protect yourself after a breach. Go to Identity-Theft.gov.

The most common types of fraud:

- Banking
- Bankruptcy
- Health
- Housing and Mortgage

- Immigration
- Internet
- Mass Marketing
- Passport and Visa
- Postal Mail
- Telemarketing
- Telephone[46]

Clark Howard, nationally syndicated radio and TV consumer expert says:

- Do not carry a checkbook.
- Do not carry your Social Security card with you.
- Buy a paper shredder.

What to do if your identity is stolen:

- Call the bank and credit card fraud department
- Call all three credit bureaus and issue a fraud alert, get your free reports and check the report again in six months
- A copy of your drivers license to each agency in order to register an affidavit
- Contact authorities via certified receipt request
- Contact local police, Social Security Administration, and all creditors
- Contact fraud units of credit bureaus and add a victim's statement stating: "My ID has been used to fraudulently apply for credit. Call me at this number to verify all applications."
- Get new cards, new passwords, have old accounts closed at customer's request
- File a police report and get a copy
- Notify FTC 877-FTC-HELP
- Cancel and get a new savings/checking accounts
- Do not pay any bills connected to the fraud
- Do a credit freeze to limit damage[47]

Keep a close watch from all angles—insurance companies, consumer purchases, including vehicles, contractors, even professionals. File a complaint with the major agencies for any deceiving, false marketing, services and products, or any matter that you are questioning. (At the least, just call and inquire.)

You have rights as a consumer and the agencies below take your complaint very seriously. They will direct you to the proper agency that deals with your complaint, via mail.

- Your state's Attorney General, AG
- Your local Better Business Bureau, BBB
- Your state's Insurance Commission, NAIC
- Your local Consumer Affairs
- Your local Child/Adult Protective Services
- Your local Office of the Aging
- Your local Department of Social Services
- Your local Police Department
- Your local Fire Department
- Your local Chamber of Commerce
- State Professional Licensing Board

IS IT IN YOUR BUDGET?

The Masterplan to Success. Stay organized, disciplined, and focus on the task at hand. You are cunning and creative. You will do what it takes to succeed. While others are out spending their money, you see things much differently. You will be the one who thinks of investing and purchasing rental properties for cash flow, but most importantly, the one that helps others. Your strategy is to win.

What is it going to take? Are you ready to tighten the budget?

Create a system that works best for you, something as simple as the envelope system, yet so calculating, will keep you on track.

There is something intriguing about running cash through your fingers, it is what "choices" feel like, and no one controls the situation better than you do. Pick and choose your budget items. **Check all that apply:**

Housing

❏ Rent/Mortgage
❏ Home Association/Condo Fees
❏ Property Taxes
❏ Storage Garage/PO box
❏ Yard/Garden supplies/Equipment/Repair
❏ Maintenance/Yard service
❏ Pool chemicals/Maintenance
❏ Pest/Termite control
❏ Security system
❏ Home-improvement projects
❏ Home repair/Maintenance
❏ Carpet/Window cleaning
❏ Dry cleaning/Drapes/Bedding
❏ Housekeeper
❏ Appliances/Grill
❏ Furniture/Rugs
❏ Furnishings/Decorating/Lamps
❏ Heater/Air Conditioner/Fans/Humidifier
❏ Cookware/Utensils
❏ Iron/Ironing board

Utilities

❏ Heating: Oil/Gas/Electric
❏ Propane/Firewood
❏ Water/Water softener
❏ Garbage/Sewer/Dump

❑ Telephone: Landline/Cell
❑ Cable/Internet/Satellite

Transportation

❑ Car/Bus/Motorcycle
❑ RV/Boat
❑ Gas
❑ Repairs
❑ Maintenance/Oil changes/Tune up
❑ License/Registration/Inspection
❑ Parking/Tolls
❑ Tires/Brakes

Insurance

❑ Homeowner/Renters
❑ Car/Motorcycle/Boat/RV
❑ Life
❑ Disability
❑ Long-term care
❑ Health
❑ Pet
❑ Warranty

Household

❑ Groceries
❑ Toiletries
❑ Laundry
❑ Pets/Toys/Grooming/Training/Licenses
❑ Vet expense
❑ Computer/Hardware/Software
❑ Blinds/Curtains

- ❑ TV/TV Stand/Radio
- ❑ Luggage
- ❑ Tools/Vacuum

Health

- ❑ Co-pays
- ❑ Prescriptions
- ❑ Dental X-rays/Cleanings
- ❑ Vision exam/Glasses/Contacts
- ❑ Alternative health
- ❑ Supplements
- ❑ Remedies

Personal

- ❑ Makeup/Skin care
- ❑ Jewelry
- ❑ Clothes/Shoes
- ❑ Work/Uniform/Shoes
- ❑ Haircuts

Entertainment

- ❑ Vacation/Lodging/Airlines
- ❑ Subscriptions
- ❑ Dining out/Movies
- ❑ Tobacco/Alcohol
- ❑ Concerts/Sports/Events
- ❑ Hobbies/Sports/Gym
- ❑ Shopping

Memberships

- ❑ Gym

- ❑ Country Club/Golf
- ❑ Church
- ❑ Organizational
- ❑ Professional dues
- ❑ Auto club/AAA
- ❑ Sports
- ❑ Warehouse BJ's/Sam's club/Costco

Credit/Loans

- ❑ Credit cards/Visa/Mastercard/American Express
- ❑ Personal loan
- ❑ Car payment
- ❑ Child support
- ❑ Alimony

Caretaking

- ❑ Child care
- ❑ Elder care
- ❑ Babysitter
- ❑ Pet care

Education

- ❑ Tuition
- ❑ Books
- ❑ School supplies
- ❑ Tutors
- ❑ Workshops/Seminars/Speakers

Financial

- ❑ Charity/Donations/Contributions
- ❑ Tax preparation

- ❏ Retirement savings
- ❏ Investments
- ❏ Emergency funds

Miscellaneous

- ❏ Holidays/Gifts/Wishlist[48]

It is a dual win for both the Warrior and Savvy Kid. Without the finances, one cannot survive. Help is minimal and levels at poverty. The fight is real and there are many in the world today who are unable to maneuver life due to lack of funding. It is now understood early on that the focus is to strategize financially for you will fulfill your dreams and prepare for the long term, setting aside the lure of instant gratification.

"To create the life you want now and in the future, you have to become the master of your cash flow today."

~ Al Zdenek

Take your financial assessment[49]:
http://alzdenek.com/assessment-a/

With a mission to *improve lives through financial education*, Clearpoint, a Division of Money Management International, is an education-focused agency and part of the largest nonprofit, full-service credit counseling agency in the United States. A range of tools, calculators, quizzes, e-books and videos at clearpoint.org, as well as free courses on financial topics are offered[50]. https://www.clearpoint.org/resources/

Chapter 3

3D LIFE DIMENSIONS: STRONG BODY, SHARP MIND, FOREVER SOUL

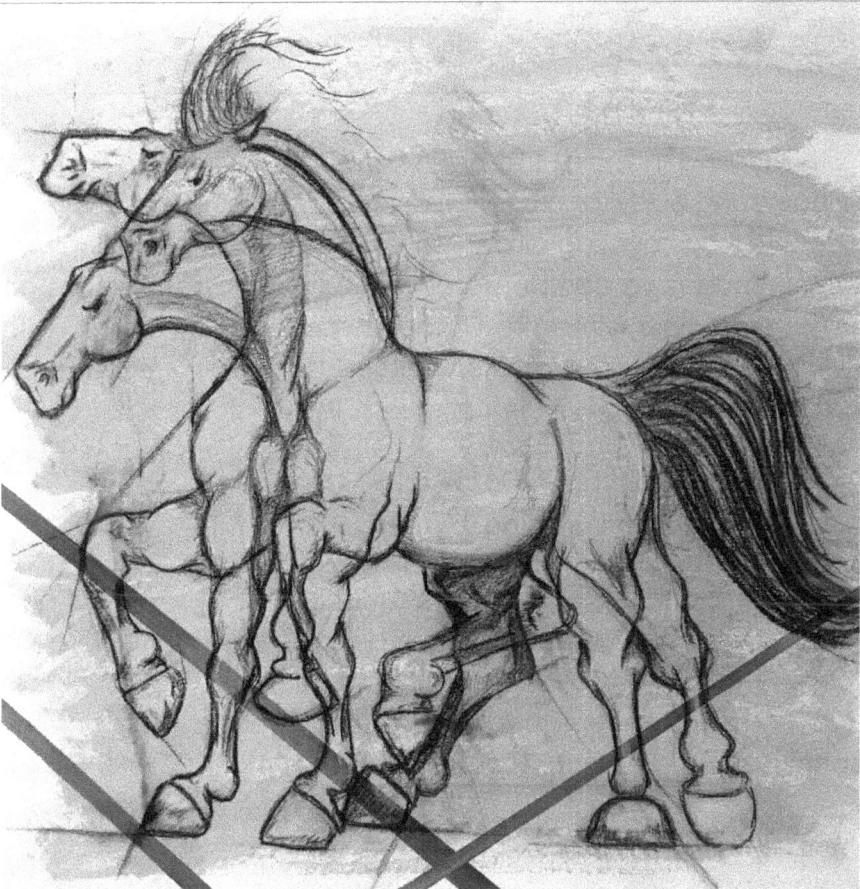

Artist Alisa Chmielinski

The vision of a leader is only to conquer, he will never accept defeat, and will build with the strength of Hercules until he can no longer speak. For the weight of surprise is on his shoulders.

A warrior believes the ultimate sacrifice is life, so he recites with all his might,

---

"Keep your friends close and your enemies closer."

~Sun Tzu

With the end in mind, the course must be maintained. Sharp mind, strong body, and a forever soul. You will succeed. Survival is secured by covering all angles. If one area fails, the troops will be summoned to compensate for the weakness. There are no barriers to your strength. Proceed and build yourself with confidence, and pull others with you. Together is excellence and there is no room to settle for less. The mission is:

"No man left behind."
"No child left behind."

The dimensions of life teach the meaning of who we are and when it is understood, weakness disappears. Excuses are no longer accepted and answers are demanded in place. Surviving relationships and being in the realm of a positive sphere brings meaning to our lives.

YOUR LIFE DIMENSIONS

Life could be viewed as a multi-dimensional battleground and the level of balance in all areas of your life will dictate at what point you will advance in achieving your goals. If you're spiraling out of control in any area of your life, a balance will have to be maintained before you can move on. Who you are, what you want, and what you will become brings you to today. Your environment, circumstances, and happenings have kept your eyes wide open so now, the path you take will be your decision and yours alone. Will you allow yourself to experience a higher level of satisfaction, enjoy the comforts of life and when successful, help pull others up to do the same? **Are you in the top ten?**

1. Do you consider yourself to be well-rounded?
2. Do you maintain control in all areas of your life?
3. Do you know who you are?
4. Do you know what you want?
5. Do you know how to get there?
6. Are you respectful to others?
7. Do you care about others?
8. Are you responsible?
9. Can you make the right decision the first time?
10. Do you believe in a higher up, something other than yourself?

Power, control, and integrity belong to you. The Circle of Wellness is the balance of life.

Do you possess the magic eight dimensions?

1. Social. Creating a support system, using good communication skills and having meaningful relationships.
2. Emotional. Accept your feelings and enjoy life despite its disappointments, frustrations, and stress.
3. Spiritual. The search for meaning and purpose in human existence, a personal matter involving values and beliefs that provide a purpose in our lives.
4. Occupational. A balance between work and life.
5. Environmental. Our interaction with nature and taking action to protect the world around us.

6. Intellectual. Engaging in creative mental activities to expand knowledge, skills, and help others to discover their potential for sharing their gifts with others.
7. Physical. Physical activity, exercise, and healthy eating. Build muscular strength, and endurance and cardiovascular strength, endurance, and flexibility.
8. Financial. Satisfaction with current and future financial situations. Live within your means and manage your finances for the short and long term[51].

Take charge and find out where you are at in the circle of wellness[52]: https://www.takingcharge.csh.umn.edu/

WHAT IS YOUR PERSONALITY?

The making of who you are begins to tell your story, so, who are you?

Characteristic patterns evolve from biological and environmental influence, thinking, feeling, and behaving. Personality embraces mood, attitude, and opinions expressed in interactions with others.

Free personality testing is available at[53]:
www.16personalities.com/free-personality-test

The information is meant to inspire personal growth and improve understanding of yourself and your relationships. It is a belief that the more people are aware of strengths and weaknesses related to their personality traits, the better and more understanding this world will be for everyone.

Five aspects of personality: Mind, Energy, Nature, Tactics, Identity.

1. Mind - shows how we interact with our surroundings:

- Introverts prefer solitary. They are exhausted by interaction and sensitive to external stimulation.
- Extroverts prefer socialization. They are enthusiastic and energized.

2. Energy - determines how we see the world and process information:

- Observants are down to earth, practical, and focus on what's happening.
- Intuitives are imaginative, open-minded, curious, and focus on the future.

3. Nature - determines how we make decisions and cope with emotions:

- Thinkers focus on objectivity, use logic over emotions and hide their feelings.
- Feelers are sensitive and emotionally expressive, empathetic, and cooperate.

4. Tactics - reflects our approach to work, planning, and decision-making:

- Judgers are organized, thorough, decisive, predictable, and prefer structure.
- Prospectors are flexible, keep options open, and spot opportunities.

5. Identity - shows how confident we are in our abilities and decisions:

- Assertive individuals are self-assured, even-tempered, and refuse to worry.
- Turbulent individuals are self-conscious, sensitive to stress, and are eager to improve, perfectionists.

What type are you?

The different roles determine your goals, interests, and preferred activities. For example:

- Analysts are independent, open-minded, and imaginative.
- Diplomats are empathetic, cooperative, and imaginative.
- Sentinels are practical, hard-working, meticulous, and traditional.
- Explorers are spontaneous, have quick reaction, and are masters of tools.

Strategies - show your preferred ways of doing things in achieving goals:

- **Confident Individualists** prefer doing things alone, are self-confident, and know what they are good at.
- **People Masters** seek social contact, express their opinions, and are confident in their abilities.
- **Constant Improvers** are quiet perfectionists and success driven.
- **Social Engagers** are sociable, energetic, and success driven[53].

Which one are you?

Type A - The Go-Getter. Hard-driven, competitive, and overachievers. They like to be in charge and be in control. In my field of work, this is the patient who is lying in bed, just suffered a heart attack and is on the phone, still doing business.

Type B - The Calming Influence. Known as grounded and have a calming peace about them. Social and highly sensitive. Very grounded and carry an aura of warmth about them. It takes a lot to get them unsettled.

Type C - The Perfectionist. Known as detail-oriented. They like things controlled and stable and are reliable. A lover of routine and having a set lifestyle. Known for having your back in a tough situation.

Type D - The Existential One. Known to be slow and easy paced. They seek security, respect and acceptance of others. Sensitive and may be isolated. Great at giving advice, and will never give up[54].

TWILIGHT ZODIAC

The 12 signs of the Zodiac give us great insight into our day to day living as well as the many talents and special qualities we possess. You can discover a great deal about yourself through reading about your Zodiac sign. Your sign is a powerful tool for understanding yourself and your relationships.

The four elements give you a feel of the psychological make up: fire, water, earth, and air.

Fire - Aries, Leo, Sagittarius
People born under this sign are driven and need to express themselves. Faith and enthusiasm are the driving forces. The flame can be a flicker or a raging flame can make them

temperamental. Passionate, impulsive. Forgive and forget quickly. Self aware and you want them on your team as you strive for greatness.

Water - Cancer, Scorpio, Pisces

People born under this sign are known to be in touch with their emotions and those of others. They can possess a higher sense of empathy. Sensitive and compassionate. They understand the motives and needs of others and will help you grow and support you.

Earth - Capricorn, Virgo, Taurus

People born under this sign are practical and cautious. They are "real" and down-to-earth. Loyal friends, they will never let you down.

Air - Gemini, Libra, Aquarius

People born under this sign are brilliant and witty, stars in their own right. Sense of freedom makes them spontaneous and unpredictable. Social, eloquent, and thinkers. Rely greatly on the power of their minds.

The Zodiac signs and Astrology form the basis of almost every story and myth that we know, including those mentioned in numerous religious texts. The map to everything that ever existed and to what will ever exist is literally written in the stars.

Which Zodiac sign are you?

Capricorn - The Goat December 22nd - January 19th
Fairness is crucial, great leaders. Realistic, bossy, and stands for the truth at all cost. Resilient, sensitive, and gentle. Ambitious, disciplined, and patient.

Aquarius - Water January 20th - February 18th
Seeks the truth, mental explorers. Observes and learns.

Brings everything to the point of truth and reality. Intelligent, energetic, and full of brilliant ideas.

Pisces - 2 Fish February 19th - March 20th
Magical thinking and will mold their personality to suit who they are with. Creative, focused, and dedicated. Talented, compassionate, and sensitive.

Aries - The Ram March 21st - April 19th
Energetic and the strongest sign of the Zodiac. Ready to take on any challenge or battle that comes their way. Excellent at getting things started. Optimistic and generous.

Taurus - The Bull April 20th- May 20th
Determined and strong. Always give a helping hand. Kind, dependable, and caring. Understands the material world. Prepared to endure the long run.

Gemini - The Twins May 21st - June 20th
Serious and sunny at the same time. Thinks quickly and needs a lot of entertainment. Inspires and you will have a lot of fun and laughter. Spirited, fast, adjustable, and smart. Communication is their biggest asset.

Cancer - The Crab June 21st - July 22nd
Love being at home and push others emotionally. Greatest strength is compassion. Trustworthy. Looks after others they care about.

Leo - The Lion July 23rd - August 22nd
King of the Zodiac. Fun and charismatic. Loves drama. Confident. Determined, loyal, warm, and childish nature. Respectful.

Virgo - The Maiden August 23rd - September 22nd
Perfectionist, sense of humor, down to earth, generous, and

have attention to detail. The most intelligent of the Zodiac. Analytical and deep. Greatest strength is their mind. Healers.

Libra - The Scales September 23rd - October 22nd
Love of all things even and balanced. Harmonious and comforting and their clothes look perfect. Tact, fineness, and responsibility. Balanced.

Scorpio - The Scorpion October 23rd - November 21st
If you cross a Scorpio, expect to feel the pain of revenge when you least expect it. Teaches others to think before acting, act honorably, kindly and with compassion. Creates peace and quiet for a deep connection. An intensity of emotion and depth of feeling is incredible and one of their greatest gifts. Greatest strength is sensitivity.

Sagittarius - The Archer November 22nd - December 21st
Loves to party. Likes to explore, enjoy new experiences, and has curious ways and tends toward infidelity. Optimistic and sincere. You will want them as a friend[55] [56].

PURPOSE AND DIRECTION TO SUCCESS

The universal human and highly personal experience touches us all. A connection to something bigger than ourselves. Spiritual practices show evidence of improvement of health and well-being.

Often the inward reflection directs your focus and quiets the mind. Broader than religion, the two are related, and both may offer questions and answers about the infinite, provide support during emotional crises, and invoke a sense of awe, wonder, and reverence. Some find that Spiritual life is intricately linked to the association with church or meditation.

You must have a free and clear mind to make the right decisions. The savvy have the power and balance to make the right decision the first time for they know about self, others, and their surroundings.

Why is Spirituality important?

- Increases compassion
- Increases empathy
- Helps you overcome hardships
- Helps you make better choices
- Helps you treat your body with kindness
- Helps you avoid unhealthy behaviors
- Longer life
- Less likely to smoke and drink
- Less likely to commit crimes
- Less likely to be involved in violence[57]

WHAT IS SPIRITUALITY FOR YOU?

Spirituality, mentioned in the wheel of life, is considered by many to be an area of calm and balance. Here are some common responses from others:

- Spirituality is the search for meaning, purpose, and direction in life.
- Spirituality is love and connection.
- Spirituality helps to reach our life potential.
- Spirituality is the answer and truth to internal happiness and a greater appreciation of life.
- Spirituality is thirst for knowledge, experience, and adventure.
- Spirituality serves others, uplifting humanity.

Five main Spiritual Paths mentioned below:

1. Knowledge, wisdom, and insight such as study
2. Devotion, surrender such as prayer
3. Meditation, stillness such as yoga
4. Service, active selflessness such as community service
5. Energy, purification of body, mind, and psyche such as breathing and yoga[58]

Seven signs that spirituality is taking hold:

1. You take care of your body.
2. You accept and love yourself as you are.
3. You accept others as they are.
4. You are less interested in material things.
5. You become more collaborative and less competitive.
6. You let go of the need to be right.
7. You love others by putting aside judgment and criticism[59].

TONY ROBBINS' FOUNDATION

The Tony Robbins' Foundation is a nonprofit organization created to empower individuals to make a significant difference in their lives. The Foundation was built on the belief system that regardless of stature, only those who have learned the power of sincere and selfless contribution experience life's deepest joy; true fulfillment:

www.thetonyrobbinsfoundation.org/programs/youth-leadership/

There is always something you can give, whether that be your time, energy or your ideas.

The youth programs and events encourage leadership in today's youth.

Focused on empowering tomorrow's leaders, The Tony Robbins Foundation provides resources, programs and events that encourage leadership in today's youth. An opportunity for younger generations to make a difference in their communities[60].

BYRON KATIE - SPEAKER, AUTHOR, FOUNDER OF *THE WORK*

Balance of life is met with clear thoughts, and for any other scenario, will require attention in order to move toward your goals. Stressful beliefs about life, people, or yourself can be shifted and your life can change forever.

Byron Katie, founder of *The Work*, has developed a process for people of all ages and all backgrounds to trace their unhappiness. Nothing more than a pen, paper, and an open mind is needed. Katie's process shows that all the problems in the world originate in our thinking, so she offers the tool to open our minds and set ourselves free.

Instead of trying to change the world to match her thoughts about how it should be, she questioned these thoughts, and by meeting reality as it is, she experienced unimaginable freedom and joy.

Maintaining a life balance goes beyond happiness and a clear mind. Alleviating stress and creating a peacefulness can also:

- Alleviate depression
- Decrease stress
- Improve relationships
- Reduce anger
- Increase mental clarity
- Increase energy

The Judge-Your-Neighbor Worksheet available at TheWork.com asks four questions that show you how to identify and question your thoughts that are causing you suffering. It is a way to understand what is hurting you, and to address the cause of your problems with clarity.

1. Is it true?
2. Can you absolutely know that it is true?
3. How do you react, what happens, when you believe that thought?
4. Who would you be without the thought?[61]

TALK IT UP

It will be of the utmost importance that as a leader, unwavering communication skills have been mastered. Orders will be given and it will be the duty of the superior to get the message across in a discreet impenetrable manner. No one must question the orders to prepare to move forward. When the command to strike is spoken, you will proceed as directed and may the best man win.

Breakdown in communication frequently has consequences such as social problems, hurt feelings, anger, divorce, and even violence.

The psychology of communication is more than just talking, it gets the message across:

- Establish and maintain eye contact. Look to get and keep the attention of others.
- Send a clear message. Use words with meaning and intention.
- Be receptive to what others say. Affirm with a nod, smile, or verbally. Use active listening.
- Wait for the other person to finish[62].

Mutual respect, caring about each other's feelings, and a two-way conversation bring people closer.

In 1971, Albert Mehrabian concluded, somewhat controversially, that only 7% of communication is verbal, 55% of communication involves non-verbal body language such as facial expressions, gestures and physical distance. The other 38% involves the tone and pitch of the voice[63].

Are you an effective communicator? Which ones below sound like you?

- ❑ Do not interrupt - apologize if it is urgent.
- ❑ Think before you speak - think how it will affect the person talking.
- ❑ Listen.
- ❑ Be neutral when someone points out your mistakes.
- ❑ Do not deviate away from the topic.
- ❑ Be confident of your ideas. This increases trust.
- ❑ Be open to feedback from the other person and give honest feedback.
- ❑ Use the right communication method and location. Privacy may be needed[64].

THE ROYAL TREATMENT

Who says chivalry is dead?

Were you taught to be a gentleman and/or a lady?

Such a feeling of respect when your partner opens the car door for you and when your partner extends their arm so you may walk hand in hand.

The Golden Rule: Do unto others as you would have them do unto you.

Courtesy is based on civility, kindness, and consideration.

Are you mindful of others when in their presence, home, or around their possessions?

Good manners will open more doors, charm more acquaintances, and make more memorable first impressions:

1. Use "please," "thank you," and "excuse me" always.
2. Wait your turn.
3. Be generous with compliments and stingy with criticism.
4. Listen to your child when they speak to you, even if you've heard it before.
5. Do not discipline your child in front of others.
6. Do not correct any child, other than your own, on his manners, and always do that privately.
7. Be clear about what you expect.
8. Be consistent.
9. Do not give in to temper tantrums.
10. Do not lose your temper.
11. Admit when you are wrong, offer an apology when you owe one.
12. Let your child know when a discussion has become a decision.
13. Words can hurt, do not hurl them about and use as weapons.
14. Respect your child's privacy and boundaries. Knock first.
15. Do not impose your ideology, and respect those who have an ideology that is different than yours.
16. Agree to disagree.
17. Give credit where credit is due.
18. Hold the door.
19. Lend a hand.
20. Be a good sport.
21. Be a gracious loser and a generous winner.

22. Give more than you are asked.
23. Do not take more than you need.
24. Leave a place cleaner than you found it.
25. Do not respond to rudeness with rudeness.
26. Winning is not the only thing, and nice guys do finish first[65].

It is never too soon to begin or too late to catch up.

SOCIAL ETIQUETTE:

1. Be on time.
2. Never show up empty handed.
3. Hold a conversation.
4. Never gossip.
5. Address others by their name.
6. Use the cell phone only when urgently needed.
7. If you are not sure how to answer a rude question, smile and change the subject.
8. Graciously change the subject when needed.

TABLE MANNERS:

1. Keep elbows off the table.
2. Napkin goes on your lap.
3. Use the flatware, starting with the one farthest from the plate.
4. Do not talk with your mouth full[66].

THE INTRIGUING MYSTERIOUS TERM - RELATIONSHIP

The Warrior relates to those around him, he is supported by his soldiers, and he gives support with his unfaltering direction. He is a Protector and will go to the greatest lengths to maintain course without defeat. The Savvy Kid maintains balance with relationships of his fellow man. He supports and protects, guides and educates, and he extends his hand to those in need, for he is a leader and on the path to success.

Everyone has a personal invitation, and you will be part of the story from the beginning. Exposure to relations begins at birth for without, there would be no survival. Relationships grow with time, good and bad, so the key is to build on your experiences. Build a strong foundation and respect the basics because living with another has its challenges, and learned behaviors start early. Some behaviors may need to be corrected to stay on the straight and narrow.

- Do you feel qualified to maneuver dysfunction? I promise you will come across it sooner than later.
- How will you react when someone wants to have a serious conversation?
- Will you be able to respond in a caring manner?
- Do you know what love is?
- Do you know what the foundation of relationships is?
- Do you come from a dysfunctional family?
- Can you spot the behaviors of an abuser?
- Do you love yourself enough to allow someone to get to know you?
- Can you spot the behaviors of a manipulator?
- What do you think about someone who wants to move fast?
- Are the red flags going up, but you're ignoring them?

It's just like doing battle. You need to have a strong foundation, be strong, have a plan, and be financially stable.

Some say when it is right, it is magical and others say the first three months are just the romance period and the real issues will soon start to set in. Radio host, Dr. Laura Schlessinger once said, "It takes about 18 months before you really get to know someone."

You are such an important individual, and despite all your learned behaviors and circumstantial happenings in your life, the decisions are yours now to flourish, succeed, and fulfill your goals and dreams. Relationships are a necessary part of life because everyone needs to feel loved, and the expectation is not one of perfection because there is no such thing, but, staying on the straight and narrow path applies to all relationships, work, friendships, family, and romance. These will forever hold your peace:

- Mutual Respect
- Trust
- Honesty
- Support
- Fairness/equality
- Separate identities
- Good communication
- A sense of playfulness/fondness

Do your relationships bring more happiness than stress?

Signs of a Healthy Relationship:

- Self-care and self-esteem independent of each other
- Respect each other
- Maintain family/friend relations
- Have separate activities
- Express yourself to one another without consequences
- Feel secure
- Take interest in each other's activities
- Violence free
- Trust and Honesty
- Give and take

- Resolve conflict fairly

Signs of Unhealthy Relationship:

- Put others first and neglect self
- Feel pressure to change who you are
- Feel worry when you disagree
- Feel pressure to quit activities
- Have to justify your actions
- Arguments are not settled fairly
- Yelling or physical violence
- Control or manipulate
- Controls what you wear or criticizes your behaviors
- Not spending time together
- No common friends or lack of respect for your friends
- Unequal control of food, money, home
- Lack of fairness and equality[67]

10 Truths to keep close to your heart:

1. Successful relationships take work by sharing what is going on in your hearts and heads.
2. You can change yourself, not your partner.
3. Arguments stem from your own fear or pain.
4. Understand that men and women are different and celebrate the differences.
5. Honor each other, respect and cherish.
6. Anger is a waste of time.
7. Get regular tune-ups; workshops, couples' getaways.
8. Become and stay best friends.
9. Be responsible for your own happiness.
10. Give what you want to get[68].

Validating, understanding, and accepting what others say shows others that you are on their side. When you accept, you show unconditional love, which is ultimately what keeps people and relationships together.

HAVE YOU EVER LOOKED INTO THE EYES OF A CHILD?

"If unsure, just look into the eyes of a child, they are the driving force of something we all once believed in."

~Robin Ann Burnham

Have you ever looked into the eyes of a child? Affirmative is the response; every time you looked into the mirror when you were little. There was no escaping it. Hopes, dreams, and fantasies may have been your reality.

Some of us grow to want to carry on our own family, which will then position you into a different realm. You become the protector, the strength, the decision maker, the financier and the psychological warrior who holds it all together. You must be prepared to make split-second decisions, because you hold in your hands someone else's life.

What do you get from a child who depends on you? Unconditional love. Unwavering love even when you falter, the total acceptance of imperfection.

Prepared for parenthood or unexpected, if you choose to take on the task you will not be sorry. Parenting is an experience that fills an emptiness for some and for others, it is an opportunity to give.

The toughest, most fulfilling job on earth is parenting, so if you are going to do it, then do it right. The way you interact with your child and how you discipline, will influence them for the rest of their lives. Children crave a sense of structure to make them feel safe.

PARENTING TELLS YOUR STORY, PERSONALITY CHOOSES YOUR STYLE

Suddenly the focus changes course from yourself to another, Warrior mode sets in. You are now the Parent and Protector and everything you do and every decision you make will set the path of success for your child. You are the tool to your child becoming safe and balanced, for it is you who teaches right from wrong. You will never give in, never give up, and your laser-beam strategy puts a life-long plan in place. Every child must know how to care for themselves, survival at its best.

Your style of parenting shows who you are and how you care for your child. It is a reflection of you, the one that raised a Savvy Kid.

Which style are you? **Check below:**

❑ **Authoritarian (Strict)**
Focus on obedience, punishment over discipline.
Follow the rules without exception. "Because I said so."
Child may become aggressive, focus on their anger toward parents.
Higher risk for low self-esteem because their opinions have not been taken into consideration, not valued.

❑ **Authoritative**
Maintain a positive relationship with your child, open communication.
Parent explains the reasons behind the rules, and enforce rules.
Parent takes child's feelings into consideration.

Children are most likely to become responsible adults who feel comfortable expressing their opinions.
Children are happy and successful, good decision makers.

"Authoritative Parenting is widely regarded as the most effective and beneficial style parenting style for normal children."
"This type of parenting creates the healthiest environment for a growing child, and helps to foster a productive relationship between the child and parent."

~Developmental Psychology at Vanderbilt

❏ **Permissive (Indulgent)**
Do not enforce rules, "Kids will be kids."
Parent sets rules and does not enforce them.
Parent only steps in when there is a serious problem.
Parent takes on a friend role instead of a parent role.
Child struggles academically, behavioral problems.
Child does not appreciate authority and rules.
Low self-esteem and a lot of sadness.
Higher risk of health problems.

❏ **Uninvolved (Neglectful)**
Provide little guidance, nurturing, or attention.
Expect children to raise themselves, neglectful.
Child has low self-esteem, do poorly in school, behavior problems, and rank low in happiness, no trust.
Child has a hard time forming relationships.
Child lacks self control, and is less competent[69] [70] [71]

"Neglectful parenting is one of the most harmful styles
of parenting that can be used on a child."
"Neglectful parenting is damaging to children,
because they have no trust foundation with their
parents from which to explore the world."

~Developmental Psychology at Vanderbilt

LOVE YOUR FOOD

Fuel is needed for energy or the weakness will set in, so keep
your nutrients close.

"Thy body is your temple and shall protect you
with all its might."

-Robin Ann Burnham

The nutrients of life come at some cost, if only everything were
equal, fair, and affordable. Circumstances do arise and
sometimes make the good untouchable. In addition, the evil
temptations of the oh-so-delicious sweets can sway your
thoughts.

- Are you overwhelmed with all the specialty diets?
- What kind of protein should you take and how much
  every day?
- Would you consider a band-aid surgery to lose weight in
  place of portion control and walking?
- Do you read calories and ingredients when you buy
  food?
- Do you have a sweet tooth?
- Are your clothes getting tight?

- Do you eat due to stress?
- Can you afford fresh fruits and vegetables?
- If you are a vegan, are you eating enough protein?
- Do you have symptoms of celiac or eat gluten free?

CARLY JOHNSTON:

I had the pleasure of talking with a Registered Dietitian Nutritionist who specializes in weight management and wellness, Carly Johnston, MS, RD, LDN. I had just finished taking a Body Pump class at Gold's Gym in Norton, MA, when I noticed a table outside one of the offices. It had a bowl of apples and muffins, and, of course, I chose to take one of the muffins. Not only did it have a great taste, it met some of those sweet cravings.

Carly doesn't believe in diets and likes to encourage her clients to develop sustainable lifestyle changes that work for them. Carly feels strongly that one size does not fit all when it comes to weight loss and uses a personalized approach for every client to help them set realistic goals to conquer each week. I asked Carly to send some information that would benefit you, see below:

Organic *versus* NON-ORGANIC

Are organic foods healthier than non-organic foods?

No, organic does not mean the food is healthier, it just means that is meets the USDA's criteria for how foods are grown, handled and processed. Organic farming practices work with the natural patterns of the environment to optimize growing conditions for specific crops and they use organic chemicals that do not harm the earth.

Do organic foods look different?

Organic produce may not be uniform in shape and size and may have blemishes, compared to the seemingly flawless non-organic produce.

What about pesticides?

Organic farmers use specific insect traps, disease-resistant plant varieties, and beneficial microorganisms or "bugs" to protect their crops. Conventional farmers use pesticides to prevent mold, insects, and diseases from damaging their crops.

What about food additives?

Organic foods are free of preservatives, artificial sweeteners, colorings, artificial flavors and monosodium glutamate (MSG). Non-organic foods have safe levels of these ingredients per the FDA.

Should I buy all foods organic?

Not necessarily. Organic foods can be expensive, so just getting the fruits and vegetables in your diet is the most important. If you are interested in exploring some organic foods, follow the rule of the Clean Fifteen and the Dirty Dozen (see sidebar). The Clean Fifteen are foods in which you can buy non-organic. The Dirty Dozen are foods that are best to buy organic, because you eat the skins.

Bottom Line:

If you can't afford to buy organic, don't. When possible, buy fruits and vegetables that are in season. Wash and scrub foods before you eat them to eliminate as much pesticide residue as possible.

New England
NUTRITION

76

New England
NUTRITION
ADVISORS LLC

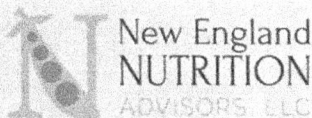

Grocery Shopping Tips

1. Start with a list: Before you go, make your meal plan for the week, including snacks. Cruise your pantry and look for items you already have to save time and money at the store. Create a list of the remaining items. Try to put the items in categories (produce, canned, meats, etc.) to make the trip as quick as possible.

2. Don't go hungry: Make sure you go to the store after a meal or snack. The last place you want to be when you're hungry is the chip and cookie aisle in the grocery store. Having something in your stomach will help you avoid straying from your list.

3. Use the nutrition facts label: This is your key to making healthy choices. Try to avoid something because of a label on the front of the product. Make an educated decision based off of these recommendations:

Look for more of these:	Look for less of these:
Fiber	Saturated fat
Vitamins A, C, E	Trans fat
Calcium	Sodium
Potassium	Cholesterol
Magnesium	Ingredients
Iron	

4. Be selective when buying organic: For most people, purchasing 100% organic foods isn't economically feasible. Sticking to the "dirty dozen" and "clean fifteen" can help keep expenses down while minimizing your intake of pesticide exposure.

Dirty dozen: (buy organic) Strawberries, spinach, nectarines, apples, peaches, pears, cherries, grapes, celery, lettuce, bell peppers, potatoes

Clean fifteen: (safe as non-organic): Onions, avocados, sweet corn, pineapples, mango, sweet peas, asparagus, kiwi fruit, cabbage, eggplant cantaloupe, watermelon, grapefruit, sweet potatoes, sweet onion

New England
NUTRITION
ADVISORS, LLC

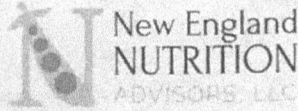

Diet and Nutrition Tips

Diets:

- Avoid diets or pills that claim to burn fat or cause excessive amounts of weight loss
  - If it sounds too good to be true it probably is
- Another red flag – detoxes or cleanses
  - Our bodies have a liver and kidneys that take care of any "detoxing" we need.
- Crash diets and very low calorie diets don't work to reduce weight in the long term
  - They slow your metabolism and can cause rebound weight gain once normal eating patterns resume

Recommendations:

1. **Drink plenty of water:** Aim for at least 64 oz. of water per day. Often times we misread hunger signals for thirst. Staying hydrated can also help prevent water retention. To meet his goal, carry a water bottle around with you and refill throughout the day.

2. **Eat 3 protein-containing meals every day:** Eating 3 meals per day will keep your metabolism revved and give you energy to get through your day. Avoid skipping meals as this can slow your metabolism and can lead to a binge at your next mealtime. An ideal plate should be ½ vegetables, ¼ protein and ¼ grains or other carbohydrates. Make sure there is a source of protein at every meal to help keep you full! That means saving large pasta dinners with no sources of visible protein for special occasions.

3. **Eat 2-3 PLANNED snacks:** The word planned is key. Instead of grabbing a box of crackers and mindlessly munching, have a measured or portion controlled snack. Some ideas are a yogurt with 2 tablespoons of granola, apple with a string cheese, or a banana with 2 tablespoons of peanut butter. Ideally you should be eating something every 3-4 hours.

4. **Take your time while eating:** It can take up to 15 minutes for your stomach to tell your brain you are full. Taking small bites and putting your fork down every few bites can help you recognize that you're full. Before going up for seconds, wait 5 minutes and if you are still hungry have an additional serving of vegetables or lean protein.

5. **Think before you eat:** Before you have an unplanned snack ask yourself if you are truly hungry or just bored. If you are truly hungry and it's only been an hour or two before your last meal/snack, grab some veggies from the fridge to snack on.

6. **Have healthy foods readily available:** Have raw veggies cut and in sandwich bags, hard cooked eggs, string cheese, measured nuts, or pieces of fruit ready to go. You are less likely to reach for a less healthy option when those are in front of you. Try to avoid bringing your trigger foods into your house if at all possible. If that isn't possible keep them in a separate cabinet away from your healthier options.

7. **Log your foods:** Some find it helpful to log their foods in an app such as *MyFitnessPal*. This adds another dimension of accountability that can help you take a second look at what you have eaten that day and stay within a healthy range of calories. It's also fun to look back at weekly weights to see how far you have come! *MyFinessPal* sends you coupons to Under Armor if you log in for a certain number of days.

8. **Get moving:** Even if you don't have time to go to the gym or do an organized exercise routine, try to stay moving throughout the day. Taking the stairs whenever possible, parking away from the building you're walking to or taking your dog for an extra walk can all add up to extra calories burned,

Carbohydrates: Carbohydrates are your body's main fuel source. Glucose is readily available while glycogen is a storage form of glucose. Your brain needs glucose to function – studying for an exam, powering through to meet a deadline, daydreaming about your next vacation. When our body is in dire need of glucose it will call upon liver or muscle cells to break down glycogen into glucose – ie. Marathon runner.
   o Sources: Plant foods (fruits, fruit juice, vegetables, grains, legumes), dairy (milk and milk products), sweets (cakes, candy, cookies, soda, sugar)
   o Not all carbohydrates are created equal
      o Choose whole grains – contain the whole kernel, less processed, nutrients remain in the food product, contain much more fiber.
      o Look for fiber on the label – 25-38 grams daily recommendation. Helps with colon health, brain health, microbiome, B-vitamins and blood sugar control.
      o Pair with protein or fat
      o Minimize processing: 74% of processed foods contain added sugar.
      o Limit sugary beverages: All day sipping leads to a constant sugar intake = constant influx of insulin = weight gain. Choose seltzer, water, decaf tea (unsweetened)
   o RDA women: 6 tsp (25 grams/d), men: 9 tsp (38 grams/d)
   o High Fructose Corn Syrup: Created in 1970, coincidentally increase in obesity started in 1970. Made in a lab. Genetically modified. Cheaper than table sugar, toxic to liver.

Protein:
- Recommendation 0.8 grams/kg body weight for most healthy adults.
  - 1 oz protein = 7 g protein
  - 1 g protein = 4 calories
- Our bodies can only process 15-25 g protein at once – protein powders providing more than that per serving gives more strain on your kidnesy and expensive urine.
  - If continuing to use protein powder, consider splitting serving size in half

Fat: An essential source of energy for our bodies. They support healthy growth, protect our organs, keep our bodies warm, help absorb fat soluble vitamins, produces important hormones.
- Not all fats are unhealthy – different fats can have different effects on heart health and cholesterol in our bodies.
  - Choose unsaturated fats instead of saturated fat:
  - Olive oil   Soybean oil
  - Canola oil   Corn oil
  - Peanut oil   Sunflower oil
  - Safflower oil   Walnut oil
  - Sesame oil   Flaxseed oil
  - Avocados   Nuts and seeds
  - Peanut butter   Fatty fish
  - Omega 3's: useful in reducing inflammation, heart disease, stroke risk.
    - Found in fatty fish (salmon, herring, mackerel), flaxseeds, walnuts
- Eating foods that contain saturated fats raises your risk of heart disease and stroke by increasing the level of cholesterol in your blood
  - Butter, lard, cream, cheese, poultry with skin, whole milk dairy products, coconut oil, fried foods, baked goods
- Trans fats: Formed through a process called hydrogenation.
  - Points of unsaturation are saturated by adding hydrogen molecules to increase shelf life and improve textures. Associated with higher risk for cardiovascular disease
    - Sources: cakes, cookies, donuts, deep fried foods, crackers
    - Label: partially or fully hydrogenated oils
- There are 9 calories for every gram of fat. This makes it more energy dense than carbohydrates (4 kcal/g) and protein (4 kcal/g). Consume in moderation!
  - 25-35% of calories should come from fat, no more than 5-6% should be from saturated fat.

HEALTHY FATS

Choose These:

Cooking Fats:
Avocado oil
Canola oil*
Corn oil
Olive oil
Peanut oil
Safflower oil
Walnut oil
*may be linked to Alzheimer's Disease

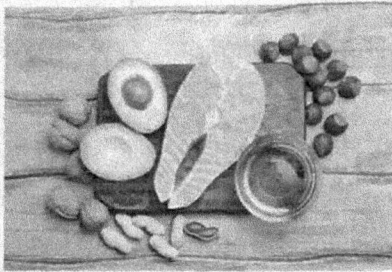

Poultry:
Skinless chicken and turkey
90-95% lean ground

Red Meat:
Loin cut
Round cut
Choice grade
Select grade

Dairy
Fat Free
1-2%
Low-Fat

Omega-3's
Salmon, Mackerel, Sardines
Walnuts
Flaxseeds
Chia seeds
Grass-fed beef

Limit These:

Coconut oil
Palm oil
Butter
Stick margarine
Fried foods
Whole milk dairy

Avoid:

Lard
Shortening
Hydrogenated oils

New England NUTRITION ADVISORS, LLC

If you would like to contact Carly[72]:
Carly@nenutritionadvisors.com (508) 942-7756

POWER UP

Power up, energize, and build strength. You will be powerful, respected, and mentally unbreakable. You will move forward because you are superior. You have what it takes to be everything, a higher level of understanding to begin with the end in mind. Your goals are attainable, and never underestimate he who is driven with an unbeatable force, a force from the wild. Knowledge is power, may the best person win.

Eating breakfast has been linked to a lower risk of obesity, diabetes, and heart disease. Replenish your blood sugar to power your muscles and brain.

Carbohydrates are your body's main source of energy. Complex carbs have staying power, you feel fuller longer and fuel your body throughout the day, stabilizing your blood sugar levels:

- Whole grains
- Fruit
- Vegetables
- Beans[73]

Protein is essential for building and repairing muscles:

- Poultry: chicken and turkey
- Red meat: beef and lamb
- Fish: salmon and tuna
- Dairy: milk and yogurt
- Legumes: beans and lentils
- Eggs[74]

Fruits and vegetables are rich in fiber, vitamins, minerals, low in calories and fat.[75]

Unsaturated fats help reduce inflammation, a primary fuel for aerobic exercise:

- Nuts
- Seeds
- Avocados
- Olives
- Oils, such as olive oil[76]

Before exercise fuel:

- Bananas
- Berries, grapes, orange
- Nuts
- Nut butter
- Crackers
- Pasta
- Low-fat yogurt[77]

Pre-Workout Tips:
Your muscles use the glucose from carbs for fuel. Protein improves muscle recovery, increases strength and lean body mass, and prevents muscle damage. Fat helps fuel your body for longer, less intense workouts.

It is recommended to consume a full meal 2-3 hours before your workout. Choose foods easy to digest to prevent stomach discomfort.

A good rule of thumb is to eat a mixture of carbs and protein prior to exercise.

The American College of Sports Medicine recommends drinking 16-20 ounces of water at least 4 hours before exercise and 8-12 ounces of water 10-15 minutes before exercise.

Not fueling up before exercise is like driving a car on empty.

Post-Workout Tips:
Getting in the right nutrients after exercise can help rebuild your muscle proteins and glycogen stores. It also helps stimulate growth of new muscle.

Studies have shown that ingesting 20-40 grams of protein seems to maximize the body's ability to recover after exercise.

A post workout meal with both both protein and carbs will enhance glycogen storage and protein synthesis. Consuming a ratio of 3:1 (carbs to protein) is a practical way to achieve this.

Eat your post workout meal within 45 minutes[78] [79]

Shakes:
- Exercise burns sugar in your bloodstream and glycogen stores in your muscles, so you have 30 minutes to restore or you will start to deplete your own muscle.
- The human body absorbs and utilizes the nutrition from a liquid much faster than from a solid (it is digested faster).
- For optimum health and sustained energy, your diet should compromise of 5-7 Low-Glycemic meals everyday consisting of nutrient-dense carbs, lean proteins and healthy fats.
- Add protein to repair or grow cells.
- Shakes should have:
  - No MSG
  - No GMOS
  - No Trans Fats
  - No added sugar
  - No preservatives
  - No artificial flavors
  - No hydrogenated oils
  - No synthetic sweeteners

○   No high fructose corn syrup[80]

DIET NONSENSE (MYTHS)

Don't believe everything you hear:

Myth #1 Lose the calories by reducing your red meat intake
Truth #1 There is nothing wrong with an occasional burger, but watch out for meat labeled "prime," it is high in artery clogging saturated fat.

- Protein keeps you fuller, longer.
- Eat lean "round" or "loin" as in top round, sirloin and tenderloin.
- Eat ground beef less than 5% fat.
- Eat two servings, or five ounces, of lean meat daily.
- Eat protein powerhouses such as fish, poultry and beans.

Myth #2 Do not eat after 8pm.
Truth #2 The body doesn't store fat and calories after a certain time.

- Choose a healthy snack like hummus or three cups of air-popped popcorn.

Myth #3 Hold steady against your cravings.
Truth #3 People are psychologically tempted by what we cannot have.

- Eat what you enjoy in moderation such as a few squares of chocolate.

Myth #4 Forget the bread.
Truth #4 Whole grain bread is fine, a complex carb that provides filling fiber.

- Refined carbs are weight-gaining such as white bread, crackers, and pastries.

Myth #5 Fat makes you fat.
Truth #5 Healthy fats help break down and absorb nutrients.

- Bad guys are saturated and trans fats are artery clogging, heart attack alley.
- Chips, crackers, fried food, butter, fatty meat.
- Good guys are unsaturated, mono, poly, and omega-3s. Fish, nuts, seeds, olive oil. Healthy fats help break down and absorb nutrients vitamin A, E and beta-carotene in fruits and vegetables.

Myth #6 Avoid fast-food drive-through.
Truth #6 Healthy is okay.

- ★ Grilled
- ★ Single serving
- ★ Reduced fat dressing

Stay away foods:

- ★ Cheese
- ★ Mayo
- ★ Creamy sauces
- ★ Fried
- ★ Double or super-sized

Myth #7 Stick to light beer.
Truth #7 You'll be more satisfied with one beer you like than two watered down versions.

- ★ Your body converts alcohol to acetate, your body burns it instead of fat for energy, slows the metabolism and halts weight loss.

Myth #8 100-calorie snack-packs will not curb the appetite.
Truth #8 Healthy 100-calorie snacks can satisfy your hunger cravings.

★ 15 almonds
★ 10 cashews
★ 3/4 cup blueberries
★ 15 chocolate covered raisins
★ 6 wheat crackers with 2 teaspoons peanut butter[81]

Great tips from Registered Dietitian Nutritionists:

1. Eat Whole plants: Beans, lentils, quinoa, brown rice, vegetables and fruits.
2. Eat more than one food group, if you are still hungry after eating a piece of fruit Combine carb and protein (at least 2 food groups) together to keep you fuller, such as an apple with peanut butter.
3. One meal will not change your health, so make it a point to eat more healthy, choosing whole grains, beans and fish over processed foods.
4. Increase fiber intake. It keeps you full - 5 grams or more of fiber per serving.
5. Stop worrying about the fat or calories and eat simple whole foods.
6. Stay away from sugar, drinks and juices, which are associated with obesity, type 2 diabetes, and heart disease.
7. Do you love nuts? They are loaded with magnesium, and vitamin E. Almonds help with weight loss.
8. Coffee is "A-OK," drinkers live longer, with reduced risk for Parkinson's and Alzheimer's diseases.
9. Fatty fish like salmon is loaded with omega 3, lowers dementia, depression and heart disease.

10. Sleep is a must, lack of can throw your hormones out of whack, and weight gain.
11. Digestive health is improved with probiotics and fiber.
12. Water is your friend, drink it before meals, it can burn calories.
13. Meat is a great protein, so do not burn it or overcook it, you will lose nutrients.
14. Stay away from bright lights before bedtime, it disrupts the hormone melatonin.
15. The sun vitamin D3, improves strength, bone, and lowers risk of cancer and depression.
16. Extra virgin olive oil is the healthiest fat of all, fights inflammation.
17. Lifting weights keeps you strong.
18. The worse of all fats is trans fat, do not even look at it, and run when you see it.
19. Herbs and spices: Ginger and turmeric are anti-inflammatories.
20. Belly fat causes the most problems, cut carbs, eat lots of fiber and protein (check with your doctor).
21. Stay away from diets, eat healthy, and walk.
22. Eat eggs, the yolk is the most nutritious but high in cholesterol[82] [83]

KEEP IT STRONG

Have you ever seen someone in great shape, muscular and lean, and do you wish you were in better shape?

Weak muscles open you up to mistakes - falls, injuries and disability.

Strength training, dumbbells or barbells can get you going. Ever hear of Les Mills exercise programs? Body pump classes?

Start with light weights and gradually increase, do 8-10 reps = 1 set, up to 3 sets, muscles should be fatigued. If not, then the weight is too light. Rest between sets, 1 to 3 minutes. Muscles need to rest for at least 48 hrs, replenish energy and grow. Switch up the routine, muscles grow accustomed fast.

Weightlifting offers balance, energy, flexibility, but it starts to diminish after age 30. Studies show 60-year-olds have the same opportunity to build muscle and reduce fat as younger people do.

Baseline should be 150 minutes per week of moderate exercise. Two to three days of cardio, alternate with 2-3 days of weight training. Stay away from weight lifting two days in a row. Follow a day of lifting with a day of cardio. Thirty minutes/day of exercise, if you can swing it. Low weight, high reps.

Tips:

- Do not spend the following day on the couch.
- Always do a 5-10 minute warm-up, brings blood flow to tight muscles.
- Do each exercise properly.
- Do not work through pain, it is your body's warning to stop[84].

Walking or raking leaves can help prevent or delay age-associated heart disease, diabetes, high blood pressure.

Exercise improves memory in older adults. Exercise reduces risk of breast and colon cancer, kidney stones, fights depression, and improves sleep. Low impact exercises are recommended for age 40 and over. When a person exercises, endorphins are released, a natural pain-killer, relieves stress and improves sleep[85].

Delayed muscle soreness is the pain and stiffness felt in muscles several hours after unaccustomed or strenuous exercise. The soreness is felt most strongly 24 to 72 hours after the exercise, then subsides and disappears up to seven days. This soreness typically is not felt at rest. The soreness can be reduced or prevented by gradually increasing the intensity of a new exercise program[86].

SWEAT SMART

Rehydrating with exercise is of the utmost importance, but so are the benefits of a great workout with a big sweat. For some, this is what gets you to come back a second time.

It's more than a muscle workout, chemicals in your brain are stimulated and produce endorphins that act as natural painkillers, sometimes helping to soothe out soreness.

Wash your face after a good sweat, after the pores open they release dirt and grime onto your skin.

Some experts consider a super sweat session a detox, flushing the body of system-clogging substances like alcohol, cholesterol, and salt.

The great mood controller, so if your feeling negative, turn it around fast with a great sweat out.

The medical benefits continue, perspiration contains a naturally occurring antimicrobial peptide called dermcidin, proven to fight dangerous pathogens.

Sweat evaporation helps prevent overheating.

An absolute positive for some, regular exercisers sweat out salt and retain calcium in the bones vs. going into the kidneys where kidney stones form.

The norm is to replenish with water when exercising, but if sweating profusely, and exercising more than one hour, then it is recommended to drink a sports drink. For longer endurance exercising, electrolytes should be replaced.

Sodium is the number one mineral lost in sweat, and one must not forget about chloride, potassium, magnesium, and calcium. Watch for low sodium - hyponatremia, muscle cramps, headaches, nausea, fatigue, thirst, and confusion, just to name a few.

The hotter and more humid the conditions, the more likely you will need electrolyte replacement. Drinking too much water can also dilute your sodium. Avocados, sweet potatoes, and yogurt are rich in electrolytes[87].

GOLDEN TIPS

Gold's Gym reports that four one-minute bursts of activity at peak levels is as beneficial as 20 minutes of low-to-moderate activity:

- Run up and down stairs.
- Take a quick jog around the block.
- Jump rope.
- Stationary bike pedaling[88].

Core is known as the torso and functional movement is highly dependent on this part of your body. Lack of a strong core will predispose you to injury. The major muscles of the core reside in the area of the belly, mid and lower back, and peripherally include the hips, shoulders, and neck.

The core is responsible for posture and support, balance and stability. Activities of daily living are dependent on strong core muscles such as lifting, pushing, standing and sitting[89].

Tips to help prevent sports injuries:

- Warm up and cool down. With your workout, keep it simple for 5-10 minutes.
- Wear proper gear.
- Wear shoes that fit properly, are stable, and absorb shock.
- Use the softest exercise surface you can find. Run on flat surfaces
- Gradually increase your activity level
- Do not bend your knees more than halfway when doing knee bends
- Do not twist your knees when you stretch. Keep your feet as flat as you can.
- When jumping, land with your knees bent.
- Do not overdo it.
- Use proper form
- Drink plenty of fluids. Avoid caffeine and alcohol.
- Work out in early am or late pm with air conditioning on hot or humid days.
- Work out indoors on windy or cold days.
- Know the signs of hypothermia and hyperthermia. Seek medical attention immediately.

Hyperthermia symptoms are: headache, dizziness, nausea, faintness, cramps, palpitations. Skin may feel moist and cool. Rest in a cool place, drink plenty of fluids, sponge off with cool water, and seek medical attention when needed.

Hypothermia symptoms are: shivering, slow speech, sleepy, pale, cold hands and feet, and anger. Move to a warm area, wrap in warm blankets, warm fluids, do not rub legs or arms, do not use a heating pad, do not warm in a bath, and seek medical attention.

Pain is your body's way of warning you that something might be wrong. If you experience a sharp pain in your muscles and/or joints, stop exercising and see your doctor[90] [91] [92].

Symptoms of sport injuries:

- Sudden, severe pain.
- Swelling.
- Not being able to place weight on a leg, knee, ankle, foot, or ankle.
- An arm, elbow, wrist, hand, or finger that is very tender.
- Not being able to move a joint as normal.
- Extreme leg or arm weakness.
- A bone or joint that is visibly out of place.

Types of sports injuries people encounter per the National Institute of Health (NIH):

- Achilles tendon injuries, connects the calf muscle to the back of your heel
- Dislocations, an abnormal separation in a joint where two bones meet
- Fractures, a break in a bone
- Knee injuries
- Ligament tears, a band of tissue that connects the ends of bones together
- Rotator cuff injuries, located in the shoulder
- Shin bone pain, known as "shin splints" -pain that shoots along the shin bone on the front of the lower leg
- Sprains, an overly stretched muscle
- Strains, a twisted or pulled muscle
- Swollen muscles, swollen and sore muscles
- Tendon tears, a cord of tissue that connects muscles to bone

When should you see an MD for an injury? If you have pain, swelling, or numbness that prevents you from putting your weight on the area.

Doctors first treat sports injuries with R-I-C-E:

- Rest, reduce your activity and rest the injured area.
- Ice, apply ice to the injury for 20 minutes, four to eight times per day. Do not place directly on skin. Wrap in a towel first before to the injured area.
- Compression, put even pressure on the painful area to help reduce swelling.
- Elevation, put the injured area on a pillow at a level above your heart. Call your doctor or seek medical attention[93].

You have become the Savvy Warrior, a leader of survival, balance, and wellness. Your foundation is built with an inner strength so strong that even Hercules is unable to move. You are a financial strategist with an understanding of time and life management. Frugal with the spending, a log is maintained of all expenses coming in and going out. Your life's dimension has come full circle for you know who you are and with a sharp mind, know how to get there. Your forever soul and spirit is what motivates and propels you in a forward motion toward success. Your sound split-second decision-making abilities will be tested soon, for the battle is on and there is no doubt that your survival skills will come into play.

CHAPTER 4

THE BIGGEST BATTLE –
LIFE'S SURVIVAL GUIDE

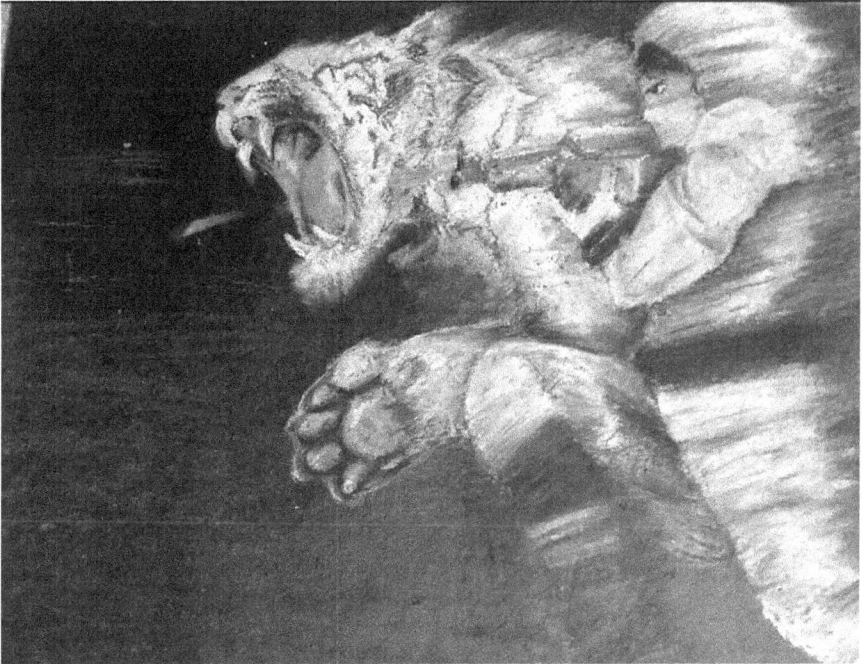

Artist Alisa Chmielinski

The battle is on. The foundation is strong, finances are in place, and your strength is unshakable. Your intuition is a keen sense and you can smell something off a mile away. Leadership takes a step forward and the thought of backing down never crosses the mind.

You live by a code: "No Man Left Behind. No Child Left Behind."

Time has become reality now, the call for engagement has been heard. The years of building, now come to fruition. Your foundation is uncrackable like walls of steel armor and your mind control is as sharp as a laser focus. Your special force vision foresees the risks and prepares for the ultimate deceptions. You have prepared and strategized for what seems like a lifetime already and now, the call to action has been placed, your strength shows no weakness. You will fight until the end until the enemy relinquishes control. You trained for this day, you have the know-how to avert any crisis that presents itself, and you have the characteristics of a warrior, so proceed and do not stop. Rise to the occasion and feel the warmth of the light because the win is an arm's length away.

BREATHE THE BASICS

The Basics of survival. Prepare for any surprise that comes around the corner, listen to your intuition and follow your instincts, it could mean life or death. You will conquer for you are the most aware.

1. **Oxygen** is the most important of all needs. So very unforgiving when depleted, that, 3 minutes without, deterioration begins. The amount of oxygen you inhale varies with the atmospheric pressure. High altitudes like Mount Everest can have a dangerously low level of partial pressure oxygen.

2. **Water** is the most essential component. You have about three days before deterioration begins. The thirst begins, then fatigue, headaches, and nausea.

3. **Food** keeps you going, and without it, you have about three weeks to survive, maybe a little longer. You will depend on fat reserves with lack of food intake, move onto the glycogen stores in your liver, and lastly the breakdown of the muscles. After all that, the beginning of the end. The fatigue, then apathy, listlessness, dry skin, and massive swelling in the abdomen area.

4. **Shelter** and **Protection** help keep the elements of nature, heat, cold and criminal or animal attacks away. Fire is one of the oldest methods to keep animals away, and locks or alarms may keep attackers away. Extreme fluctuation of temperatures may cause hallucinations or confusion.

5. **Sleep**. You require about seven to nine hours of sleep every night. Sleep deprivation becomes symptomatic after 24 hours of no sleep with headaches, then, after 72 hours, is mental impairment and spatial deterioration. The sleep deprivation record is 11 days. It is dangerous and can literally kill you, so it was removed from the *Guinness World Book Of Records*[94].

SMARTER THAN TROUBLE

Carry a first-aid booklet with you, for you will never regret it. It may just pull you through the surprise visit of trouble, showing you are the smarter one.

So you have been asked to go for a trail bike ride, hike on foot, camping, or you are lost in the woods:

Do you know your survival tips?

Do you know the essentials needed to pack?
Do you trust your partner to bring the right items?
Do you know your survival techniques?
Can you make it out alive?
Will you starve?

Prepare Ahead:

The thought process a survivor must have, "I will survive no matter what!"

Air

Water: keep a filter in your bag. Approx 2 liters per person each day and double on hot days.

Water purification tablets: The safest sources of water is rainwater collected on a tarp. Boil stream water for 10 minutes.

Food: protein and meal replacement bars work well for energy, dried fruit, nuts.

Clothing and shoes: loose clothing and layer. Hat or Bandanna. Poncho.

Shelter: Always make sure there is a way out.

Plan: Map and money in a waterproof bag - make a list of contacts, places and leave a copy behind. Make someone aware of your departure plan and when you expect to be back.

First-aid kit and medications: keep a three-day supply with you. Antihistamine, sunburn cream, triple antibiotic, aspirin, ibuprofen, hydrocortisone cream, lip balm, calamine lotion.

Waterproof matches, firestarter and windproof lighter: you may need to boil water to purify, signal with a fire, or cook to survive.

Stick to the trail and know the regulations: If caught in a flash flood, move to high ground.

Essentials:

Flashlight
Ham radio, whistle
Knife
Axe
Rope
Compass
Binoculars
Hygiene products - toilet paper
Solar cellphone and battery charger
Camping pot
Sunscreen
Insect repellent with DEET
Multi-tool
Mummy sleeping bag and an inflatable ground mat
Fishing line
Candle
Signal mirror
Pencil and paper[95]

Lightning: a bolt can be 5 miles long, 100 million volts, and generate a temp of 50,000 degrees. The sound takes five seconds to travel one mile.

Remember the phrase,

"When thunder roars, go indoors"

~CDC, Centers for Disease Control and Prevention

Lightning Safety Tips:

- Do not lie on concrete floors or lean on concrete walls, lightning can travel through any metal wires or bars in the concrete.
- Stay away from metal and get rid of any metal objects.
- Run for cover, a metal-roof car, just do not touch the metal.
- Stay away from trees, lightening loves tall objects.
- If you are out in the open then squat down, on the balls of your feet, head between knees and fold hands over head. Do not lie down, lightning causes electric currents along the top of the ground that can be deadly over 100 feet away.
- Avoid water. Do not bathe or wash dishes.
- Avoid electronic equipment: computers, laptops, game systems, washers, dryers, anything connected to an electrical outlet.
- Avoid corded phones.
- It is safe to use a cell phone if it is not connected to a charger plugged into an outlet. A cordless phone is okay to use.
- It is safe to touch someone that is hit by lightning.
- Call 911 immediately![96]

HIKING IN BEAR COUNTRY:

Stand strong like a Warrior, if you run, you lose. If a bear attack pursues play dead, face down with hands over head. Learn and play the game of life.

Precautions:

If you smell something dead or see birds circling overhead, avoid the area. Bears do not like you near their food areas.
Pack your food tightly, even food bits attract.
Bear signs - tracks, scratches, and markings on trees.
Do not wear scented lotions or perfumes.

Face to Face:

Do not run, you will not outrun a bear. Stand calmly.
Talk to the bear and slowly wave your arms up and down to show him you are a human. No eye contact.
If the bear approaches, stand your ground, when he stops charging then back away slowly.
If he attacks then play dead by lying face down with hands over your head. Same position if he rolls you over.
Grizzlies attack out of defense.
Black bears are less aggressive but predatory in nature, fight back if he attacks.
Use your bear spray[97].

EMERGENCY AND DISASTER PLANS:

Preplan an evacuation route.
Family and Pet emergency plan
Obtain emergency information from FEMA (Federal Emergency Management Agency) FEMA.gov
Wireless Emergency Alert public safety system (WEA) weather.gov Sign up for alerts
Disaster in a foreign country DisasterAssistance.gov

Smart Traveler Enrollment Program (STEP) for local updates step.state.gov
Learn about conditions that may affect safety and security abroad 1-888-407-4747[98]

ADVENTURING WITH YOUR DOG

According to Lisa J. Godfrey in Adirondack Life magazine, 2018 Guide To The Great Outdoors Issue:

Dogs are considered to be "Man's Best Friend," just short of being human. For you are their master and they count on you to protect. Someday you may need them to save your life. Together you are stronger than one.

Critical basics for your dog:
    Must know basic commands: sit, stay, down, heel, leave it, up, drop it.
    Carry a leash, water, and food for dog.
    Must have a collar with your name and contact number.
    Current dog tag (if required in your area).

Hiking:
    Work up to longer hikes for their paw protection and endurance
    A dog should never carry more than 10% of their body weight
    Harness with handle to assist him
    Treats: hard-boiled eggs or cheese

Paddling:
    Introduce the boat on dry land and teach him to sit and lie on the bottom
    Lifejacket for master and dog
    Yoga mat on bottom, so dog does not slip

Camping:

    Keep dog near you at all times

    Pad or sleeping bag for dog to sleep on

    Dog food kept in bear canisters

    Reflective collar or clip on light

First Aid Kit:

    Bandana for a muzzle if dog is injured, they can snap if in pain

    Blanket for shock

    Nose pliers for extractions

    Duct tape

    Insect repellent

    Benadryl

    Dog comb

    Paperwork for vet, vaccine records, nearest vet and contact/location info

Treat Dog Troubles:

    Wounds - Generally not recommended to wrap a bandage around a limb of a dog, can compromise circulation.

    Heat stroke/exhaustion - Place a cool wrap around head or paws. Do not use ice

    Bites/Stings - Seek vet help if you see hives or swelling[99]

PETS, PLANTS, AND POISON

So trusting and yet so toxic, just like the apple Snow White ate. The hidden secrets of life can poison you and your pets, may you be smarter than the unknown. Knowing who to call is the key to survival.

Poison Control 1-800-222-1222 Poisoncontrol.org Plant Booklet "What's Poisonous and What's Not"
Free Download - Poison Control Checklist

Animal Poison Control 1-888-426-4435 ASPCA.org

Pet Poison Helpline 1-800-213-6680

"Guide To Pet Safety" Petpoisonhelpline.com

Tips/Warnings:

Keep pets away from chocolate, grapes, raisins, currants, macadamia nuts, garlic, yeast dough, onion, alcohol, avocado, chocolate, coffee and caffeine, citrus, coconut and coconut oil, milk and dairy, chives, raw/undercooked meat, eggs and bones, salt and salty snack foods, xylitol, an ingredient sometimes found in gum, candy, baked goods and toothpaste.

Empty mop buckets (cleaning products), animals will drink any liquid when thirsty.

Mothballs are toxic.

Automotive and windshield fluid are toxic and life threatening.

Aspirin can be fatal for animals along with other medications.

Nicotine/tobacco may cause seizures and death.

Alkaline batteries can burn your pet's mouth and stomach. Choking hazard if stuck in the stomach or intestines: surgery is a must.

Petroleum products - gasoline, mineral spirits, can be absorbed through the skin and burn your pet.

Paint: lead-based can cause lead poisoning.

Pesticides, Insecticides, and Herbicides are toxic.

Toxic Plants:

> Acorns and wild mushrooms
> Easter lily
> Philodendron
> Pothos plant
> Bracken fern
> Cocoa bean mulch
> Sago Palm
> Tulips
> Aloe
> Poinsettia
> Azalea
> Marijuana
> Oleander
> Amaryllis
> Chrysanthemum
> Pine Christmas Tree
> English Ivy………………. just to mention a few!

Holiday Time:

> Christmas tree water can contain bacteria.
> Choking hazard from tinsel, ribbons, tree needles.
> Poinsettia is not toxic but the sap cause mouth irritation and rashes

Holly leaves are prickly and can cause injury. The berries are poison.

Flea products - use according to directions and some are weight based.

Pet toys - rawhide swells, cow hooves can splinter and puncture the stomach and intestines.

Common household - modeling clay, medications, Ethylene Glycol (Antifreeze)

Keep 3% Hydrogen peroxide available, it is used to produce vomiting Do Not Use unless directed by the vet or Poison Control

DON'T PANIC

Choking and poisonous hazards can produce instant fear in another and children love to put everything and anything in their mouths. Remaining calm, cool, and collected, consider taking a Basic Life Support class, this technique could save a life:

Poisons:
Medications
Nicotine
Chemicals
Rhododendron
Holly berries
Pokeberries
Fruit pits, seeds, and leaves
Iris
Daffodils
Lily-of-the-valley
Mistletoe
Morning glory...........Just to mention a few

Non-toxics:
African violet
Begonia
Christmas cactus
Dandelion
Impatiens
Marigold
Petunia

Poinsettia (may cause irritation)
Spider plant
Wild strawberry
Wild mushrooms.........Just to mention a few

Non-Toxic Choking Hazards:

Chaulk can block the breathing if it gets stuck in the throat

Pencil is not real lead, it is graphite.

Markers felt tipped and water soluble are not usually harmful.

Erasers are a choking hazard.

Glues: Elmers is non-toxic. Krazy Glue is non-toxic but may cause skin surfaces to stick together, including eyelids and cause eye injury.

Paint: (water- based) latex, tempera, and poster paints may irritate skin or mouth. Swallowing large amounts may cause vomiting.

Birth control pills are non-toxic.

Antacids

Zinc oxide or Lanolin - (diaper cream) a lick or swallow is not dangerous but more may cause nausea, diarrhea, vomiting.

Petroleum jelly, if swallowed may cause a cough or lung symptoms for 24 hours and it may cause diarrhea.

Talcum powder is dangerous if inhaled. It can damage the lungs and cause death. Keep away from children.

Diaper wipes and liquid may cause mouth irritation, may upset stomach. Some wipes contain alcohol and that will drop a child's blood sugar ********* Call Poison control 1-800-222-1222**

Diaper product in eyes: pour room temperature water across the eyes for 15 minutes.

Potting soil

Vermiculite

Styrofoam

Silica Gel (packet in shoe boxes): Non-toxic choking hazard.

Foreign Objects Swallowed:

Coins add up close to 80% needing surgical removal.

Button batteries are extremely dangerous. **Go to the ER. Call The Battery Ingestion Hotline 1-800-498-8666.**

Objects stuck in the esophagus (food tube) or throat. Symptoms to watch for: chest pain, coughing, gagging, vomiting, refusing to eat, drooling. **Call 911, Go to the ER, Call Poison Control 1-800-222-1222.**

Accidents happen, we understand. Make the call.

Two ways to get help:

1. 1-800-222-1222
2. Web POISON CONTROL online tool (https://triage.webpoisoncontrol.org) and download the app to your phone from Google play or App Store

First aid for Poisonings poison.org/actfast

If the individual collapses, has a seizure, has trouble breathing, or can't be awakened, call 911.

Before you seek help from the Poison Control, whether by phone or online, there are some quick first-aid measures that make a difference if accomplished within seconds to minutes of the poison exposure:

Swallowed poisons: if burning, irritating, or caustic and the person is conscious, not having convulsions, and able to swallow, drink a small amount of water or milk immediately. **Then get help from Poison Control:** use webPOISONCONTROL to get specific recommendations for your case online or call **1-800-222-1222**.

Poison in the eye: Rinse (irrigate) the eye immediately. Every second matters. A delay could result in loss of sight. Remove contact lenses. Use lots of room temperature water and irrigate for at least 15 to 20 minutes. Adults and older children may find it easiest to hop in the shower. Wrap young children in a towel and let water from the faucet in the kitchen sink run over the eye – or slowly pour water from a pitcher. Let the water hit the bridge of the nose and gently run into the eyes rather than pouring the water directly into the eye. **Important: Irrigate for at least 15 to 20 minutes**. Encourage blinking. Use web**POISON**CONTROL to get specific recommendations online or call Poison Control at **1-800-222-1222** for help.

Poison on the skin: Rinse the skin immediately. Remove contaminated clothing first (that's clothing with a spill). Don't delay. Every second matters. Use lots of room temperature running water. For large spills, adults and older children may find it easiest to hop in the shower. Use mild soap to remove material that sticks to the skin. Important: Rinse for at least 15 minutes. Use web**POISON**CONTROL to get specific recommendations online or call Poison Control at **1-800-222-1222** for help.

Inhaled poison: Move to fresh air immediately. Stay away from toxic fumes and gases. Use web**POISON**CONTROL to get specific recommendations online or call Poison Control at **1-800-222-1222** for help.

S.O.S.

The well-known common distress code. For many, it was first learned from the movies when one draws the initials in the sand after being shipwrecked on an island.

The famous rhyme known to decipher poisonous vs. non-poisonous snakes. Remember, for this may make you smarter than them.

"Red touch yellow, kill a fellow. Red touch black, friend of Jack."

-Jack Loticus, 1982

You will meet up with a spider sooner than later, there is no escaping this one. Know which ones are dangerous. For something so small, they can fight a strong battle.

Visiting or vacationing the ocean waters, you may meet up with a jellyfish or algae bloom. Respect ocean life or feel the pain of its sting.

Prevention is worth its weight in gold.

Venomous Snakes:

Pit Vipers - requires observation for possible antivenin
    Rattlesnakes
    Copperheads
Water Moccasins (cottonmouths)
Coral Snakes - require antivenin

First Aid:

    Get away - Do they have?
    Large triangular head
    Rattle
    Black nose on red, yellow, and black bands
    Remove any jewelry near bite, swelling will occur
    Keep area at or below heart level
    Do not ice, will worsen
    Do not apply a tourniquet
    Do not cut and suck the bite site
    snakes can bite

Get to the ER, Call 911, Call Poison Control
*****1-800-222-1222 *****

Spiders:

Scorpion
    Stings cause burning, stinging pain. Wash with soap and water. Over-the-counter pain reliever. Call Poison Control.

Black widow
    Has tiny puncture wounds and has a ball-like abdomen and causes pain right away. Achiness, numbness in 1-3 hours. Cleanse area with soap and water. Go to ER. Call Poison Control. Anti-venom may be needed for a severe case. You will need a tetanus booster.

Brown Recluse

Violin markings on head - blisters, bulls eye, ulceration and necrosis, fever, chills, go to the ER. There is no antidote. May need antihistamine, antibiotic, surgery and tetanus.

Tarantula

The bite will leave fang marks and throbbing pain. Fever, nausea, and vomiting may occur. Spider hairs cause pain, redness, itching, swelling and may get into the eyes (hairs may need surgical removal) There is no antidote - cool compresses and over-the-counter pain relievers. Wash with soap and water and remove hairs with sticky tape. Call Poison Control.

Jellyfish Stings:

Rinse with sea water

Remove tentacles - apply shaving cream or baking soda paste and water, shave with razor or the edge of a credit card.

Itching - anti-itch cream and/or antihistamine, check with the pharmacist.

Pain - over-the-counter pain reliever. Check with the pharmacist.

**If stung in the mouth, eye, or genital region then go to ER
Call 911 if trouble breathing and call Poison Control
1-800-222-1222**

Red Tide and Algal Bloom:

Warm temperatures, sunlight and added nutrients cause an overgrowth or bloom of algae (red tide), a natural phenomenon producing toxins that can poison when swallowing, swimming, or inhaling the water or when eating fish. Water shades of red, brown, yellow, or green. (Summer and early Fall)

Algae may accumulate in shellfish, scallops, clams, mussels and oysters. Illness can result in:

- Neurotoxic numbness and tingling of face, hands, feet, nausea, diarrhea, vomiting. Symptoms may go away in three days without treatment.
- Skin irritation, rash, itching and nose, eye, and throat irritation.

******Call Poison Control 1-800-222-1222 ******

WebPoisonControl.org - the first online triage tool and app to provide individualized guidance for poison emergencies[100].

STORMS AND SHOOTINGS - BE READY

The battles of life continue and as the title mentions, you better be ready, for you may find yourself in the eye of the storm. You are smart, calculating, and precise. You will know what to do before it happens.

Snowstorms and Extreme Cold:

Stay off the road

Prepare for power outages - keep refrigerators and freezers closed, throw out food if the temperature is 40 degrees or higher. Disconnect appliances and electronics from the power source to avoid damage.

Refrigerators will keep the temp cold for approximately four hours

Freezer will keep temp for approximately 48 hours

Use generators outside only and away from the home at least 20 feet

Do not use gas stovetop or oven to heat the house

Check on neighbors

Check for signs of frostbite and hypothermia

Frostbite - loss of feeling and color around the face, fingers, toes numbness, white or greyish-yellow skin, firm or waxy skin. Get to a warm room. Soak in warm water. Use body heat to warm. Do not massage or use a heating pad. Seek emergency treatment as soon as possible.

Hypothermia - low body temperature. Below 95 degrees is an emergency - shivering, exhaustion, confusion, fumbling hands, memory loss, slurred speech, drowsiness. Get to a warm room. Warm the center of the body first. Chest, neck, head, and groin. Keep dry and wrapped up in warm blankets, including head and neck.

Prepare the home by caulking, insulate and weather stripping. Keep pipes from freezing.
Sign up for the emergency alert system - EAS
Sign up for the alert system National Oceanic Atmospheric Administration - NOAA
Car emergency kit - jumper cables, sand, flashlight, warm clothes, blankets, bottled water, non-perishable snacks, full gas tank.
If trapped in the car, stay inside[101].

Rip Currents/Rip Tides:

Be prepared for your visit to the ocean, the undertow can take you down:

Fast moving and powerful enough to sweep you out to sea from the Great Lakes to the Ocean's waters. Channels of water narrow with an undertow often form near beaches, piers, reefs, jetties and sandbars. Eighty percent of beach water rescues are due to riptides. Rip currents can move 8 feet per second.

Watch for the tides:
    A channel of churning, choppy water

An area of noticeable different water color
A line of foam, seaweed or debris moving steadily seaward
A break in the incoming wave pattern

What can you do to survive?
Never swim alone
Life guarded beaches only
Remain calm
Do not fight the current
Swim out of the current in the direction following the shoreline (parallel)
When out of the current, swim to shore
Wave for help
Do not enter to save someone, throw them an object[102]

Hurricane Preparedness:

Are you prepared?
If you need housing - FEMA.gov
If you need food, water, shelter, call Red Cross 1-800-733-2767
Check the weather Alerts.Weather.gov scroll down and select your state
Is the water drinkable? (Drink bottled water only)
Disaster Distress Helpline 1-800-985-5990
Financial assistance FEMA.gov 1-800-621-3362

Category 1-5:
1- 74-95 mph winds Dangerous
2- 96-110 mph winds Extremely dangerous
3- 111-130 mph wings Devastating
4- 131-155 mph winds Catastrophic
5- 155+ mph winds Catastrophic

Preparation:

The pharmacy will fill your prescriptions early in a hurricane warning.

Place financial documents in the dishwasher and lock.

Fill bathtub with water.

Emergency kits can be purchased from your local Red Cross.

Emergency Kit:

1. Water - one gallon per day per person, three-day supply
2. Food - non-perishable three-day supply
3. Flashlight
4. Battery powered radio NOAA weather radio
5. First Aid Kit
6. Seven-day supply of medications and medical items
7. Multi-purpose tool
8. Sanitation and hygiene items
9. Copies of personal documents
10. Cell phone and charger
11. Family and emergency contact info
12. Cash
13. Full protection shelter
14. Maps
15. Hand crank flashlight, radio, and charger
16. Non-electric can opener and paper products
17. Gasoline for the vehicle
18. Propane for the grill

Beware of Scams after the Storm:

Building Repair and Contracting

Assignment of Benefits Issues

Tree Service

Charity

Disaster Relief[103]

Active Shooter:

RUN. HIDE. FIGHT

Look for the two nearest exits anywhere you go, and identify hiding places

Get away from the shooter is priority

Leave your belongings behind

Help others escape

Warn others

Call 911 and describe shooter, location, and weapons

Stay quiet

Silence electronics

Lock and block doors, close the blinds, and turn off lights

Do not hide in groups

Use text, social media, or put a sign in the window to tag your location

Stay in place until police give the all clear

Act as aggressively against the shooter as possible

Recruit others to ambush the shooter

Makeshift weapons with chairs, fire extinguishers, scissors, books

Be prepared to cause lethal harm to the shooter

Throw items to distract the shooter

Take care of yourself first then help others

Apply first aid - pressure to wounds

Seek help for the long-term effects of a trauma

Flooding:

The most common natural disaster in the United States: causes outages disrupts transportation, damages buildings, and creates landslides.

Turn around, don't drown, and seek shelter fast!

Six inches of water can knock you down, and one foot of moving water can sweep your vehicle away.

Stay off bridges, they can be washed away with fast moving water.

Evacuate when told to do so.

Move to higher ground or a higher floor if you stay where you are.

Prepare:
- Check the FEMA Flood Map Service Center for flood risk to your area.
- Sign up for the emergency alert system (EAS) and National Oceanic and Atmospheric Administration (NOAA) Weather Radio for emergency alerts.
- Learn your evacuation route, shelter plans, and flash flood response.
- Gather supplies for a quick exit, and don't forget about the needs of your pets.
- Batteries and phone chargers are a must.
- Are you in a flood zone? Do you need flood insurance? (National Flood Insurance Program (NFIP)
- Are your important documents in a waterproof container? Create password-protected digital copies just to be safe.
- Protect your property. Move valuables to higher levels, declutter drains and gutters, install check valves and consider a sump pump with a battery.
- If your vehicle is trapped in rapidly moving water, then stay inside. If water is rising, get out onto the roof.
- If you're in a building and the water is rising, move to higher levels or to the roof.

During cleanup:
- Wear heavy gloves and boots, critters may be in the water in your house.
- Beware of getting electrocuted. Turn off the electricity before hand.
- Use a generator or gasoline-powered machinery outdoors only and away from windows.

Earthquakes:

Sudden, rapid shaking of the earth, caused by a break and shift of underground rock.

Higher risk areas include California, Alaska, Mississippi but can occur anywhere.

Can cause damage to roads and fires, tsunamis, landslides, and avalanches.

Drop, Cover, and Hold on! Drop to your hands and knees, cover your head and neck with your arms, find cover, and hold onto something sturdy.

Do not go outside or get in a doorway. If in a car, pull over and stop. If in bed stay there and cover your head and neck with a pillow.

Prepare:
- Secure moving items
- Have a family emergency contact set up. Know where to meet afterward in case of separation.
- Supply kit for three days of food and water, flashlight, whistle, and fire extinguisher. Medications and pet care.
- Are you in a high risk area? Do you need earthquake insurance?
- Expect aftershocks.

Wildfire:

A raging, out-of-control fire usually triggered by lightning or accidents. They spread quickly, igniting brush, trees, and homes.

Prepare:
- Have a set meeting place, a family plan in case of separation.
- Smoke alarms on every level of your home, especially the bedrooms.
- Check with your local fire department about getting a free one.
- Check alarms every month and change the batteries every year.
- Keep the yard clean, rake the leaves.
- Call 911 if you spot a fire.
- Fill outdoor tubs, pools, or garbage cans with water.
- Place important documents in your car, instead of the garage. Put the pets in the car.
- Turn all outside lights and inside lights on so the house can be seen.
- Report any post fire sparks or smoke throughout the house.
- Watch for dangling or downed lines, beware of electrocution.
- Look out for ash pits or hidden embers, you could get burned.
- Do not use faucet water.

Tornadoes:

Violent, rotating columns of air that extend from a thunderstorm to the ground. May have a loud roar like a freight train.

Winds can be intense, over 200 mph and look like funnels.

- Get to a sturdy building immediately, go to a safe room, basement or the lowest level.
- Stay away from windows, doors, and outside walls.
- Do not get under an overpass or bridge. Your safer in a low, flat area.
- Watch out for flying debris. Use your arms to protect your head and neck.

Prepare:

- Know your area risk. Midwest and Southeast are at greater risk
- Sign up for the emergency alert system (EAS and NOAA) Consider having a storm room built using FEMA criteria or a storm shelter built to ICC 500 standards. The next best protection is a windowless, interior room on the lowest level of a sturdy building.
- Cover yourself with your arms and blankets[104].

Stay Close To The Finances:

Ask yourself, "What if disaster strikes, am I prepared?" The aftermath is the vision that will set you up to prepare. Keep the cash and documents close. Use an external hard drive to backup data and back it up to a free cloud service and protect your documents with password proof management. You must be able to prove who you are. Keep your documents in a locked, fireproof, waterproof container.

Financial preparation documents to keep with you:

- ❏ Insurance documents
- ❏ Medical Records and prescriptions
- ❏ Birth/marriage certificates
- ❏ Mortgage info
- ❏ Car registration

- ❑ Passports
- ❑ Drivers license and ID
- ❑ Social Security card
- ❑ Tax returns
- ❑ Employment info
- ❑ Wills/Deeds
- ❑ Stocks/Bonds/Negotiable certificates
- ❑ Bank/Savings/Retirement accounts
- ❑ Pet medical records/ID tags/Carrier
- ❑ Recent utility bill/School registration/Government documents[105]

CARBON MONOXIDE THE SILENT KILLER

Is Your Home Safe?

- Keep fixed and portable space heaters at least three feet from anything that can burn. Turn off when you leave the room or go to bed.
- Install smoke alarms on every level of the home, inside bedrooms and outside sleeping areas. Interconnect them so when one sounds, they'll all sound.
- Make a home fire escape plan and practice every three months.
- Keep candles at least one foot from anything that can burn.
- Blow out candles when leaving the room or going to bed.
- Test alarms monthly and replace batteries when "chirping."
- Replace alarm if 10 years old.
- No smoking in bed.

Do You Know What The Silent Killer Is?

Carbon Monoxide - invisible, silent, and odorless. A toxic gas from burning fuel (gasoline, kerosene, wood, propane, natural gas)

Due to improperly operating gas appliances and exhaust:
Furnace
Water heater
Dryer
Range
Fireplace
Gas and diesel vehicles
Gas-powered machines
Wood-burning fireplaces

Symptoms:
Headache and dizziness
Fatigue and weakness
Watering and burning eyes
Nausea and vomiting
Loss of muscle control
Confusion
Stomach pain
Chest pain

Prepare:
- Install and maintain CO detectors according to manufacturer's instructions.
- Record the expiration date.
- Replace the CO detectors battery annually or when needed.
- Vacuum your CO detectors monthly.
- Have fuel-burning appliances checked by a qualified technician per manufacturer's specifications.
- Clear indoor/outdoor vents and chimneys of debris, ice and snow and a chimney serviced yearly.

- Check furnace filter monthly.
- Check flame on all natural gas appliances regularly, the flame should be blue.
- Wood-burning stove area should have adequate air supply with an open window.
- Do not idle your car in the garage even with the garage door open.
- Properly install and maintain a carbon monoxide detector.

Help:
- Evacuate the area immediately and get into fresh air
- Call 911
- Call your local fire department[106]

PROTECT YOUR ID

Alert! Alert! Alert! With the progressive nature of technology it is imperative that you as a consumer stay on top of your game. Identity theft is real and they are trying to infiltrate your devices in any way they can. Keep things clean and protected, and you will outplay the players.

CyberSecurity:

Keeping All Web-Connected Devices Clean:
- Keep free of malware and infectious risks.
- Delete unused apps, review your app permissions.

Keeping Things Secure:
- Username and passwords are not enough to protect you strengthen your accounts by authentication tools when offered.
- Secure your router password, stay away from any self identification.
- Passwords should be at least 12 characters long.

Digital File Purge and Protection:
- Copy important data to a secure cloud site or another.
- Dispose of sensitive materials.
- Delete old files, and unsubscribe to newsletters, email updates, and alerts.
- Review privacy and security settings on websites.
- Delete Social Media photos that no longer represent who you are[107].

DRIVE WITH A CLEAN SLATE

Driving can get you where you want to go faster but be prepared because it comes with a financial responsibility of maintaining and a maturity that will keep you out of trouble. Know what to do before the trouble begins, for those split-second decisions will come in handy.

Driving Safety:

Check for recalls at www.nhtsa.gov/recalls - free VIN lookup tool.

Winter stock your vehicle with a snow shovel, broom and ice scraper. Use sand or kitty litter for extra weight in case you get stuck in the snow. Jumper cables, flashlight, and warning devices such as flares or emergency markers. Blankets for the cold. A cell phone with charger, water, food, and any necessary medicine.

Summer stock your vehicle with a cell phone and charger, first aid kit, flashlight, flares and a white flag, jumper cables, tire pressure gauge, jack and ground mat to change a tire, work gloves and a change in clothes, basic repair tools and duct tape to repair a hose leak, water ad paper towels, nonperishable food, water, and medicine, extra windshield wiper fluid, maps and emergency blankets, towels, and coats.

Auto Maintenance:

Get your car serviced - tune-ups, oil changes, battery checks and tire rotations. Check for recalls

Check your tire pressure monthly when the car has not been driven for three hours or more, and check the spare. The correct pressure is found on the door pillar or doorframe or in the vehicle owner's manual. The correct tire pressure for your vehicle is not the number listed on the tire itself. Under inflation is the leading cause of tire failure.

Check for tire tread wear. The "penny test" determines when it is time to replace your tires. Place a penny in the tread with the Lincoln's head upside down. If you can see the top of Lincoln's head, your vehicle needs new tires.

Checklist:
- ❑ Air conditioning and heating
- ❑ Cooling system
- ❑ Fluid levels
- ❑ Belts and hoses
- ❑ Wiper blades
- ❑ Floor mats
- ❑ Lights
- ❑ Emergency roadside kit
- ❑ Tires
- ❑ Battery

Winter Driving Safety:

- Never warm car in an enclosed area.
- Keep tires properly inflated.
- Never mix radial tires with other types.
- Keep gas tank at 1/2 full to prevent freezing of gas line.

- Avoid cruise control on slippery surfaces.
- Look and steer where you want to go.
- Watch the weather. Let others know of your route, destination and ETA.
- Pack cell phone, blankets, gloves, hat, AAA number, shovel, food, water, candle, waterproof matches and your medication.
- Stay with vehicle if snowbound.
- Tie a bright cloth on antenna or top of the window to signal distress. Keep dome light on to help rescuers find you.
- Check exhaust that it is clear to prevent carbon monoxide poisoning.
- Run heater to take chill off then preserve fuel by shutting off.
- Accelerate and decelerate slowly to regain traction and avoid skidding.
- Margin of safety is to follow eight to 10 seconds.
- Keep the heel of your foot on the floor and use the ball of your foot to brake, firm, steady pressure.
- Try not to brake, slow down enough to keep rolling until a light changes.
- Do not power up hills, pick up speed before the hill. Do not stop on a hill.

Summer Driving Safety:

- Never leave a child alone in a car - not even for a few minutes or with the engine running.
- If the outdoor temp is in the low 80s, the temperature in the car can reach deadly levels in just a few minutes- even with the window rolled down.
- All children under age 13 should ride in the back seat.
- A child's temperature rises three to five times faster than that of an adult.

- Before you back out of a driveway or parking spot, prevent backovers by walking around your vehicle to check for children.
- Backup cameras are not full proof, objects may be out of your view but in your path.
- The bigger the car the bigger your blind spot.
- Keep your doors locked.
- Leave more distance between you and a motorcyclist (3 or 4 seconds)
  Watch for motorcyclists, bicyclists, and pedestrians. Be attentive around schools and neighborhoods where children are active.

DRIVING EMERGENCIES:

Skidding:

Remove your foot from the gas pedal. Steer where you want to go. Never slam on the brakes.

Tire Flats

Let off the gas pedal and slow to stop.

Tire Blowout

Let off the gas pedal. Do not use brakes. Hold onto the steering wheel tight and slow to stop.

Brake Failure

For wet brakes, test after going through water, if no response, pull off the road and call for help. For total failure, standard brakes pump, anti-lock brakes do not pump. Shift to low gear and apply brakes slowly. Press release button or lever to prevent rear brakes from locking. Rub the tire against the curb to try and stop. Drive off road onto dirt to try and stop.

Engine Stalls
> Brakes and steer will still work but will be hard to control. Pull off road. Call for help.

Power Steering Failure
> You can steer but it will be hard. Brake slowly. Pull off Road. Call for help.

Accelerator Stuck
> Shift into neutral and slowly brake. Pull off road. Shut off the engine and put the emergency brake on. Call for help.

Engine Overheats
> Pull off road and stop. Turn heat on high to cool engine. Call for help.

Carbon Monoxide Poisoning
> Check exhaust. Watch For a headache, dizziness, tiredness, flu-like, nausea and loss of consciousness[108]

DUI

Honor and Respect is the name of the game. Know the rules of your state.

Driving under the influence of drugs and alcohol will bring on a stiff penalty and you may just find yourself in the slammer.

It's time for some tough love. Do not get behind the wheel of a moving vehicle, if you do, you will pay the price and it will be high.

National Cost Of A DUI:
> Minimum fine= $390
> Penalty Assessment= $666
> State Restitution Fund= $100
> Alcohol-Abuse Education Fund= $50

Blood or Breath-Testing Fee= $37
Jail Cite-and-Release Fee= $ 10
Driving/Alcohol-Awareness School= $375
License Reissue Fee= $100
Attorney Fees= $2,500
Auto Insurance Increase= $3,600-$6,600
Total= $7,828 - $10,828

The first thing to go is your judgment, second is your vision, and then your coordination. Last but not least, if your already depressed, plan on going to the deep end because alcohol is a depressant.

Symptoms of alcohol overdose include mental confusion, difficulty remaining conscious, vomiting, seizures, trouble breathing, slow heart rate, clammy skin, dulled responses such as no gag reflex (which prevents choking), and extremely low body temperature.

12 oz Beer = 5 oz Wine = 1.5 oz 80 proof alcohol
Most states limit for DUI = .08 gms/100 milliliters of blood alcohol,
Or breath alcohol = .08 gms/210 liters of alcohol

A 12-ounce can of beer (about 5 percent alcohol, a 5-ounce glass of wine (about 12 percent alcohol), and 1.5 ounces of 80-proof distilled spirits (40 percent alcohol) all contain the same amount of alcohol and have the same effects on the body and mind.

On average, it takes 2 to 3 hours for a single drink to leave a person's system. Nothing can speed up this process, including drinking coffee, taking a cold shower, or "walking it off."

Blood alcohol concentration (BAC) can continue to rise even when a person stops drinking or is unconscious.

Be potential danger of alcohol overdose is choking on one's own vomit.

In most states:

Misdemeanor - fine of $1000 and up to one year in prison or both

Felony - fine up to $5000 and/or five years in prison

Manslaughter - Felony and prison time and fines

Vehicular Homicide - Felony with fines and prison time[109] [110]

MADD (MOTHERS AGAINST DRUNK DRIVING):

Drunk Driving is still the #1 cause of death on our roadways.

Every 2 minutes, someone is injured in a drunk driving crash.

Every 51 minutes, someone is killed.

2 out of 3 people will be impacted by a drunk driving crash in their lifetime.

1 in 4 drivers tested positive for at least one drug that could affect safety.

Everyday in America, another 30 people die as a result of drunk driving crashes.

300,000 incidents a day.

10,876 deaths a year.

4,300 people are killed each year due to teen alcohol use- more than all other drugs combined.

6X youth who start drinking before age 15 are 6 times more likely to develop alcohol dependence or abuse later in life.

#1 car crashes are the leading cause of death in teenagers.

1 in 4 car crashes with teenagers involve an underage drunk driver[111].

BEWARE EVIL LURKS AND IS GETTING STRONGER

As a Warrior prepares and strategizes to fight for a belief, he can focus on nothing else. He prepares for any attack, from any angle, and for the worst-case scenario and then during battle, never accepts defeat.

More today than ever, the warrior inside must be on alert status at all times. Beware and strategize prior to a happening. In appearance evil is gaining strength, but we will overcome because we are smarter and will fight harder. We will protect our children, the world we live in, and we will fight till the end. We will win the war!

ABUSE

Domestic violence and abuse can happen to anyone, do not let it be you. Watch for those red flags flying high for they are your warning signs. Trust your instincts and make your move early with a cordial pleasure to meet you and leave it at that.

Domestic violence and abuse are used for one purpose only and that is to gain total control over you.

An abuser will use fear, guilt, shame, and intimidation to wear you down.

Behavioral Signs of Child Abuse: physical abuse and neglect, sexual abuse, emotional maltreatment

- Wary of adults
- Aggressiveness, withdrawal
- Frightened of parents
- Afraid to go home

- Reports injury by parents
- Begging, stealing food
- Alcohol or drug abuse
- Withdrawal, fantasy, infantile behavior
- Reports sexual assault
- Runs away
- Unwilling to change for gym
- Learning problems
- Developmental lags, problems concentrating
- Attempted suicide
- Passive

Behavioral Signs of Domestic Violence: indirect physical abuse and neglect, psychological abuse and neglect.

- Delay between injury and treatment
- Repeated ER visits
- Hospital/doctor hopping
- Hesitant, evasive, embarrassed when describing accident
- Untreated old injuries
- History of suicidal ideations or attempts
- Psychosomatic and emotional complaints
- Fear of going home
- Fear for children's safety
- Apologizes for partner's behavior

Behavioral Signs of Elder Abuse: indirect physical abuse and neglect, psychological abuse and neglect, financial abuse, exploitation, sexual abuse.

- Reported by victim
- Brought to hospital by someone other than caretaker
- Hospital/doctor hopping
- Unexplained injuries
- Lack of concern from caretaker

- Withdrawn, fearful, agitated in presence of caregiver
- Isolation
- Family or caregiver blaming elder
- Unrealistic expectations of victim by caregiver
- Evidence of need for or reluctance to part with elders' Social Security check, other assets to provide for alternative care, even family or caregiver desire respite

Relationship Violence

Can you recognize the signs?
- ❏ The victim is afraid of their partner and anxious around them.
- ❏ The victim cuts calls short when partner is around and cuts contact with friends and family.
- ❏ The victim's partner is critical and may humiliate.
- ❏ The victim's partner forces sex.
- ❏ The victim's partner orders them around.
- ❏ The victim's partner has a temper, is jealous, bad-tempered.
- ❏ The victim is anxious, depressed.
- ❏ The victim has physical injuries.

Do you:
- ❏ Feel afraid of your partner?
- ❏ Avoid certain topics out of fear of angering your partner?
- ❏ Feel that you cannot do anything right for your partner?
- ❏ Wonder if you are the one who is crazy?
- ❏ Feel emotionally numb or helpless?

Does your partner:
- ❏ Humiliate or yell at you?
- ❏ Criticize you and put you down?
- ❏ Have a bad and unpredictable temper?

- ❏ Act excessively jealous and possessive?
- ❏ Constantly check up on you?

Abusers use a variety of tactics to manipulate you and exert their power. Red flags to be aware of:
- ❏ Dominance
- ❏ Humiliation
- ❏ Isolation
- ❏ Threats
- ❏ Intimidation
- ❏ Denial and blame

Number One Priority For Victims Is Safety

Safety Plan and Hide it:
- ❏ Documents - Marriage and Drivers license, Birth certificate
- ❏ Money, checkbook, credit cards, ATM, mortgage, car title
- ❏ Social Security card, work permit, green card, passport, visa, marriage, divorce, custody, restraining order
- ❏ Insurance papers, medical records
- ❏ Rental, lease, house deed
- ❏ School and health records
- ❏ Keys - house, car, office, friend
- ❏ Medications, glasses, hearing aids
- ❏ Personal - address book, pictures, toys
- ❏ Copies - partners green card, social security card, immigration documents
- ❏ Benefit card
- ❏ Know your escape route
- ❏ Always have an exit
- ❏ Stay near a phone
- ❏ Devise a code word
- ❏ Trust your judgment[112] [113] [114] [115]

Call The National Hotline   1-800-799-7233
TTY   1-800-787-3224
TheHotLine.org

Sexual Assault:

Sexual assault is one of the many ways an abuser maintains power and control over their victim.

Every 92 seconds, an American is sexually assaulted. Every 9 minutes, that victim is a child. Only 5 out of every 1,000 perpetrators will end up in prison.

Are you or someone you know experiencing sexual violence from an intimate partner or have questions about consent?[116]

* Call LoveIsRespect   1-866-331-9474
TTY   1-866-331-8453

Are you in need support and resources specific to sexual assault including assault that is not from an intimate partner?

RAINN is the nation's largest anti-sexual violence organization. RAINN also carries out programs to prevent sexual violence, help survivors, and ensure that perpetrators are brought to justice[117].

* Call RAINN (Rape, Abuse and Incest National Network) at 1-800-656-HOPE (4673)

Human Trafficking:

Human trafficking is defined as a situation in which an individual is compelled to work or engage in commercial sex through the use of force, fraud, or coercion. Force, fraud, or coercion need not be present if the individual is under 18 years of age.

Human trafficking has been identified as the largest human rights violation in the history of mankind.

Modern-day slavery describes the act of recruiting, harboring, transporting, providing, or obtaining a person for compelled labor or commercial sex acts.

According to a report by the FBI, four-fifths of victims were identified as U.S. citizens (83%).

The average age a teen enters the sex trade in the U.S. is 12 to 14 years of age.

- The problem is Enormous.
- The essence of trafficking is Coercion.
- The motivation is Money.
- Anyone can be a victim of Forced Labor and Sex Trafficking.
- They prey on Vulnerability, Lie, and give False Promises, Isolate, Control, Extort and Intimidate.
- Manipulate immigration status and threaten to harm family members.
- Beat, torture, and abuse.
- They do whatever they have to compel a victim to labor or prostitute.
- Prosecute the traffickers, not the victim.
- Traffickers can be stopped with vetted specialized investigative units.

Watch For The Red Flags:

- Is not free to come and go as they wish
- Under age 18 and is providing commercial sex acts
- Is in the commercial sex industry and has a pimp
- Unpaid, paid little, paid tips only
- Works excessively

- Is not allowed breaks
- Owes a large debt
- Was recruited under false promises
- High security measures exist at the work or living place
- Windows are boarded, bars on windows, barbed wire, security cameras
- Is anxious, depressed, submissive
- Exhibits fear after bringing up law enforcement
- Avoids eye contact
- Lacks health care
- Appears malnourished
- Shows signs of abuse
- Has no personal possessions
- Is not in control of their money, financial records or bank accounts
- Is not in control of their documents - ID or passport
- Is not allowed to speak for themselves
- Inability to state where they are staying
- Does not know where they are
- Loss of time
- Inconsistent stories

Does this sound like anyone you know?[118] [119] [120]

National Human Trafficking Hotline   1-888-373-7888
TTY   711

Child Abduction:

Immediately call law enforcement:
- ❑ Give the child's name, date of birth, height, weight and any unique identifier
- ❑ When was the child missing?
- ❑ What clothes did they have on?

❏ Enter child's name into the National Crime Information Center (Missing Person File) (NCIC)[121]

Gangs and Related Activities:

Can you recognize the involvement? They have their own language, graffiti, hand signs, colors, tattoos, and certain types of clothing.

Staggering statistics:
2,300 gang members under age 15 in NJ, as young as second and third grade.
46% of gang-related incidents occur on school property

Why do they join:
- Security, protection, sense of belonging
- Lack of family
- Sense of respect and status
- Living in a gang infested community
- Low self-esteem
- Financial opportunity
- Peer pressure
- Thrill seeking
- Media glorifying violence

Warning Signs:
- Admits membership
- Defiant behavior
- Grades drop
- New friends
- Calls from unknown people
- Unexplained money and jewelry
- Slang
- Flashing signs
- Graffiti
- Nicknames and street names

- Evidence of drug abuse

What can be done to prevent children from joining a gang?
- Open and frequent talk with the kids
- Athletics
- Limit exposure to violence
- Cultivate respect to others and property
- Know who their friends are
- Curfew
- Be involved in their lives[122]

MS-13:

"Kill, rape, control." That's the motto for Mara Salvatrucha, or MS-13, a transnational criminal organization dubbed "the most dangerous gang in the world."

- International criminal gang, first appeared in Los Angeles among El Salvadoran immigrants who fled the civil war.
- The word "Mara" is a term for gang." Salva" comes from EL Salvador. "trucha" is slang for clever. 13 refers to the thirteenth letter of the alphabet, or "M", which denotes the gangs allegiance to the Mexican Mafia, a prison gang.
- Prefer machetes and knives.
- Known for tattooed faces, a sign of loyalty.
- Between 1980 and 1990, the population of Salvadoran immigrants in the US increased from 94,000 to 465,000.
- According to 2008 FBI estimates, MS-13 spans 42 US states and is comprised of about 50,000 members worldwide.
- MS-13 Human smuggling efforts are focused on Sex Trafficking and Prostitution.

- In 2009 there were nine Child prostitution rings discovered in Maryland, Virginia, and the District of Columbia.
- MS-13 is one of the largest street gangs in the US.
- MS-13 has a large presence in New York, Virginia, and the Washington D.C. metropolitan area.
- MS-13 EL Salvador leaders have been sending representatives to cross into the U.S. illegally, to gain control of local MS-13 cliques and reconstitute them. They are directed to become more violent to control territory. They are involved in extorting legitimate businesses and illegal businesses such as prostitution and gambling[123] [124].

Recognize the signs for the bloods, crips, Latin kings, neta and ms-13: https://www.nj.gov/oag/gang-signs-bro.pdf

ISIS:

- An extremist movement, now pursues jihadist agenda - resources, territory, arms.
- Want to be known as Islamic State.
- They captured Mosul's central bank.
- Brought foreign fighters back to Iraq
- They are still gaining ground.
- American interests are at stake.

Signs of recruitment:
- Are they using phrases you have never heard?
- Are they avoiding typical slang?
- Have they changed the way they dress and/or groom?
- Have life-long friends been replaced or removed from their social circle?
- Are they spending more time online than usual? Are they secretive of where they are going online?

- Are they exhibiting obsessive religious behaviors like reading from the Quran in isolation?

If you suspect, what should you do?

Do not try to compete with the ISIS propaganda, they may simply revert into backdoor surfing, further alienating them from you.

Do not ban from social networks.

The key is openness with your child. Watch the videos, read ISIS updates, and discuss what is being shown. Know and understand how ISIS works. Listen to your child's views.

The child is guided by open engagement on the truth about ISIS - the stories of those that have escaped will become your best reference.

Open discussions, community support and calling on trusted specialists[125] [126].

KKK (White Supremacist):

David Cunningham, Professor and Chair of Sociology at Brandeis University (Oxford University Press, 2013) reports that isolated extremist themselves can become a breeding ground for unpredictable behavior. In the absence of a broader organization, racist violence can be much more difficult to prevent or police.

Iconic racist symbols of the KKK: white hoods, flowing sheets, fiery crosses and vigilante violence.

Today, the Southern Poverty Law Center reports active KKK groups in 41 states, although the groups remain small.

According to the USA Today, August 6, 2018 it was reported that ziploc bags filled with Ku Klux Klan recruitment flyers and candy had been found in the driveways of area schoolchildren, a suspected effort to recruit children in New York. Confirmed by the Oneida County Sheriff's Office. Beware[127]

Mass Shootings:

A gunman kills at least four victims. The majority of perpetrators are white males who act alone. Contributing factors according to Wikipedia:

- Accessibility of firearms
- Mental illness treated with psychiatric drugs
- The desire to seek revenge due to a long history of being bullied
- A wide gap between self expectation and actual achievement
- Desire for fame and notoriety
- Copycats
- Lack of government background checks

Soft Targets and Crowded Places:

Homeland Security Awareness for Soft Targets and Crowded Places has put an action plan in place to protect we the people. As much as we wish things were different today, the fact is, terrorist attacks and propaganda are real. It is our duty to protect our children, young, old and ourselves. Be ready, be alert.

Vehicle Ramming is the use of a car as a weapon to cause harm with a devastating effect. **Run. Call 911. Seek cover.**

A Chemical Attack is the deliberate release of toxins such as a gas, liquid, or solid to cause harm, injury, or loss of life. Common household and professional grade toxic chemicals can be used in an attack including nerve agents, blister agents, blood agents, choking agents, and irritants.

- Sarin is a nerve agent and Odorless.
- Chlorine is a chemical agent and smells like Bleach.
- Hydrogen Sulfide is a chemical agent and smells like Rotten Eggs. Highly toxic.
- Phosgene is a chemical agent and smells like Mown Hay.
- Phosphine is a nerve agent, a chemical agent and smells like Decaying Fish or Garlic.
- Arsine is a chemical agent and smells like Slight-fish or Garlic. Can be fatal.

Signs of chemical exposure: eye/skin irritation, twitching, choking, difficulty breathing, dizziness, muscle weakness, and loss of consciousness. Toxicity may occur through inhalation or absorption through the skin.

Indoors: Find clean air, cover nose and mouth. **Call 911.**

Outdoors: Avoid any plume or vapor cloud. Seek shelter, lock doors, close windows and air vents to block external airflow. Seal the room from outside air. Seek higher ground to avoid chemical contact that often remains at surface level. **Call 911.**

Fire as a weapon has been used consistently to cause harm to people and property. Leave the area immediately. If indoors, close the door behind you to confine the fire[128]. **Call 911.**

The Death Trap Suicide:

The cry that screamed but nobody heard, they didn't really want to die, they just wanted the feeling to stop. How many times have we heard after an unexpected suicide, that the signs were there but no one saw them or acted upon them to intervene? Maybe there was an attempt to help but it was a speeding train out of control. Sometimes it is a cover-up by the victim. Sometimes it is the beginning of the end and one instance could change its course. Is it a hormonal imbalance? Is this you? Are you numb to the fight? The reality of the subject will touch your life at some point because we all know someone, cared for someone or heard of someone that gave up the fight. Be smarter, be quicker and be stronger. You are the protector. Treat others as you would like to be treated.

Can you see the signs?

Can you hear the subtle hints?

Can you intervene quick enough?

Can you communicate and get the real answers?

Do you know someone at risk?

- Mental disorders - mood disorders, schizophrenia, anxiety, personality disorders
- Alcohol and substance abuse
- Hopelessness
- Impulsive and/or aggressive tendencies
- History of trauma or abuse
- Major physical illnesses
- Previous suicide attempts
- Family history of suicide
- Job or financial loss
- Loss of relationships
- Isolation and lack of support
- Exposure to others - internet
- Family violence
- Prison

- Ages 15-24 and over age 60

Can you see the warnings?

- ❑ Talking about harming self or no reason to live
- ❑ Looking for a way to die
- ❑ Feeling trapped or unbearable pain
- ❑ Talking of being a burden
- ❑ Increased alcohol or drugs
- ❑ Anxious, agitated or behaving recklessly
- ❑ Sleeping too little or too much
- ❑ Withdrawing or isolating self
- ❑ Rage or seeking revenge
- ❑ Extreme mood swings
- ❑ Giving away possessions[129] [130]

Get Help ASAP - As soon as possible - Tell someone.

National Suicide Prevention Lifeline 1-800-273-TALK (8255)

Bully Smully

So here we are in the year 2018 and bullying has not only brought some to their knees but has driven them to suicide.

Bullying is aggressive, repeated, unwanted power imbalance. In layman's terms we can say the brutal, relentless cruelty and demeaning abusive behavior from one person to another.

Cyberbullying takes it to the next level of online harassment, mistreatment, making fun of another while using cell phones text or emails.

Do I his a form of online harassment by making personal information public
Posting mean, hurtful comments or rumors

Nude photo sharing against someone's will

Encouraging self-harm or suicide

Bullied for being gay

Lies and false accusations

Bullied for being economically challenged

False identity profile, sometimes referred to a "Sockpuppet"

Stopbullying.gov Get Help Now Here

How To Deal With The Bully:

- Not responding will help de-escalate the bully's behavior.
- Get help and report the interactions immediately.
- Do not believe anything he says.
- File a report with the school, work and/or police.

Possible Consequences for the bully:

1. School suspension
2. Expelled from the school
3. Legal charges of harassment, stalking, identity theft or defamation of character
4. Criminal record
5. Attend counseling[131] [132]

Bullying Matrix

Type of Bullying	Parent
Physical • Hitting • Kicking • Shoving • Spitting • Hazing	**Notify** the school immediately if you find out this is happening to your child. **Request** information about the school's policy. **Follow up** to make sure administrative processes are followed.
Verbal • Teasing • Name calling • Insults • Rumors • Gossip	**Listen** to your child. **Do not blame** him/her for being targeted. **Keep track** of the bullying, including when and where it occurs, so you can provide the school with details. **Make it clear** to your child that many value him/her. **Don't** let the bully's version become your child's identity. **Monitor** your own behavior and make sure you are not modeling these.
Emotional/Non-Verbal • Exclusion • Damaging Property • Intimidating Gestures • Faking Friendship	**Emphasize** the importance of seeking out those who treat others with respect. **Be proactive** in encouraging friendships. **Find** social networks for you child outside of school; this will lessen the impact of this kind of behavior. **Alert** the school if the behavior persists. **Recognize** that this can be an indication of poor social skills or learning differences.
Cyber – Using text, email, social networks to • Spread rumors • Embarrass or humiliate • Generate "quizzes" about students • Send hurtful messages	**Help** your child eliminate the means of attack (blocking email, text, unfriending, etc.). **Contact** the service provider and school to notify them of abuse. **Understand** this type of bullying often works both ways, and hold your child accountable if he/she participates. **Discuss** the potential consequences of the permanent record that remains on the Internet.

Hooked On You The Opioid Crisis

One try might get you hooked, that was the word when I was growing up. Today its an epidemic, so what changed? The stories of overdose and death, the pictures of crystal meth smokers with rotten teeth and the aging beyond their years is gut-wrenching to see. There is no discrimination and all are welcome to try but beware that the drug of choice may be laced with your death. The drugs are laced with killer doses. The dealers and suppliers are making a profit off your suffering.

Radio show host, Sean Hannity, had a guest caller who verbalized that her daughter had passed of a drug overdose. The conversation went like this, "Since the makers know what they are putting in the drugs, and causing death, it would lead one to believe that this may be chemical warfare."

Opioid Timeline:

The timeline of the opioid addiction crisis:

1970 - Short-term pain relief opioids on the market.

1980 - Opioids being spoken of as a potentially non-addictive solution to pain.

1990 - Nationwide concern over growing untreated or poorly managed pain.

1995 - FDA approved Oxycontin the first sustained release opiate drug for the long term. Pill-mills began popping up.

1996 - The Pain Society push to view PAIN as the fifth vital sign after blood pressure, heart rate, respiratory rate, temperature.

2003 - The FDA issued a warning to the Purdue Pharmacy for misleading advertisements.

2014 - Fentanyl began entering the drug supply.

2017 - A public health emergency called to combat the crisis by US Department of Health and Human Services.

Dangerous Synthetic drugs ****** Alert Alert Alert ******

- Heroin and Fentanyl mixture
- K2/Spice synthetic cannabinoids laced with blood thinner
- Counterfeit Oxycodone with synthetic opioid fentanyl
- Yellow Opioid
- Cocaine and Fentanyl
- Grey Death several potent opioids, U-47700 (Pink), Heroin and Fentanyl
- Carfentanil animal opioid 10,000 times more potent than Morphine. Used for large animals, including elephants
- Counterfeit prescriptions laced with Fentanyl
- Synthetic Cannabinoids Cloud 9, Relax, Crown (AB-PINACA, AB-FUBINACA) used in E-cigarettes, Mojo, Spice, K2, Scooby Snax (MAB-CHMINACA, ADB-CHMINACA)
- Kratom linked to salmonella infections

Club Drugs

- GHB
- Rohypnol
- Ketamine
- MDMA (Ecstasy, Molly)
- Methamphetamine
- LSD (Acid)

Common Misused Over The Counter Medications

- Dextromethorphan (DXM) cough suppressant. Taken with antihistamines and decongestants. Called robo-tripping or skittling.

- Loperamide antidiarrheal

Commonly Abused Drugs

* Alcohol
* Ayahuasca
*Central Nervous System Depressants
* Cocaine
*DMT
*GHB * Hallucinogens
* Heroin
* Inhalants
* Ketamine
* Khat
* Kratom
* LSD
* Marijuana - Cannabis
* MDMA - Ecstasy/Molly
* Mescaline - Peyote
* Methamphetamine
* Over-the-Counter Medicines - Dextromethorphan (DXM)
* Over-the-Counter Medicines - Loperamide
* PCP
* Prescription Opioids
* Prescription Stimulants
* Psilocybin
* Rohypnol - Flunitrazepam
* Salvia
* Steroids - Anabolic
* Synthetic Cannabinoids
* Synthetic Cathinones - Bath salts
* Tobacco[133] [134]

Self-Defense:

Have you ever been in a situation where you had to defend yourself from an imminent threat?

The use of force in self-defense generally loses justification once the threat has ended. Any use of force against an assailant after that is no longer self-defense but retaliatory.

The fear of harm must be reasonable and match the level of threat in question. You must employ only enough force to match the threat and be able to stop defending when there is no longer justification. Some states require that you attempt to escape from the threat first before using force, called the duty to retreat.

Do you know your state's law about the castle doctrine? Can you use deadly force against someone who unlawfully enters your home?[135]

What would you do? Flight or Fight or Freeze?

In the face of fear or traumatic happenings, our response of flight or fight is one of survival. There is hope that with action we can survive the situation. Stand your ground and fight back, fight long enough to get away or just run as fast as you can. Your body's response reacts with a surge of adrenalin suddenly giving superhuman energy and strength to outfight or outrun any attacker. On the other hand if there is no chance of escape, you feel hopeless or overwhelmed, the freeze response may take over. Sometimes your best option is to play dead[136].

Your survival-oriented acute stress response is triggered if you assess the immediate menacing force as something you potentially have the power to defeat. Your hormones are released by your sympathetic nervous system-especially adrenaline-priming you to do battle.

If you view the antagonistic force to be too powerful to overcome, your impulse is to outrun it, and this is the flight response.

What you perceive as a dire threat, is the totally disabling freeze response. This reaction refers to a situation in which you have concluded that you can neither defeat the frightening dangerous opponent confronting you nor can you safely bolt from it. This is a self-paralyzing response, "freezing up" or "numbing out", dissociating from the here and now.

Personal Protection Tips:
- Stay calm, never show your fear.
- Stay close to the attacker, he will have a harder time hitting.
- Hit him hard, fast and first, then try to escape.
- Hit where it counts - groin, throat, thigh and stomp on his foot.
- Block the hits with your hands up.
- Push the assailant to the ground and run.
- Fight only until you can escape.
- Get back up and fight, and do it quickly[137].

The goal is to save your life.

Split-second decisions may be all you have!

Street Smarts:

The risk to your safety is high, some see only the darkness and wish you to follow. Scary times ahead means it is time to watch your back. The stakes are high and increasing but why? The increase in sex trafficking, gangs, murder, abduction, violence, bullying, abuse and assault are all to real and commanding your attention.

Evil vs. Good, both lay their cards on the table in front of you, stare deep into your soul and ask, "Which road will you travel?" The fight is on, now proceed and may the best man win.

Protect and defend, for the time may soon come. Criminals look for people who walk with their heads down, staring at the ground. So counteract with confidence, head up and eyes scanning. Now they will see you as alert and guarded.

- Spend the extra money on good locks, and steel doors.
- Insert large dowel rod stops on the windows so they only open five inches.
- Watch the body language - if you can't see the palms of the hands, they are a threat. Hands are key!
- Pay attention to details when scanning your environment.
- Use a stern tone of voice when giving commands.
- Divert and confuse.
- Take a Self-Defense training course.
- Push your opponent off balance.
- Use charm and humor, it shows a calmness, no fear, no intimidation, all while creating confusion and diversion.
- Dogs are your best friend - an early warning system. Pay attention to them!
- Put up a "Beware of Dog" sign.
    - Guard dogs bark and hold their ground and may bite
    - Attack dogs come after you
    - Chihuahuas teach that bluffing works!
- Imminent death - fight until the end.
- Use your nails - best at neck, face, eyes but beware this could be fatal.

- Have your keys ready in advance - let the keys protrude through your fingers making a fist.
- Hair Brush - break their hands, knees and head.
- Rings - punch or back slap.
- Purse - swing heavily.
- Heels - drive the heel in the top of their feet.
- Umbrella with a long metal tip - break ribs and punctures body mass.
- Cane - concealed swords, knives hidden within the cane, a secret compartment
- Teeth - bite the attacker.
- Body alarms - wear on belt, key ring, outside of purse home alarms - motion detection, flood lights, sirens and cameras.
- Interior/exterior lights should be on a timer[138].

A special Thank You to Hawk Bishop Survivalreport.org
How To Protect Yourself Like A PRO

Fraudster:

Trickery at its best. They want your personal information and your money. Double check all your transactions and trust your gut instincts. If you feel something is just not right then it probably isn't. Keep your eyes and ears wide open!

Areas of interest:

- Banking
- Bankruptcy
- Health
- Housing and Mortgage
- Immigration
- Internet
- Mass Marketing
- Passport and Visa

- Postal Mail
- Telemarketing
- Telephone

Scams:

Your wisdom and intelligence are at the highest level now. The battle is on and the evil undertow is attempting to pull you in. Your laughter will deafen the ears of those that attempt to come up against you. So foolish are they to even attempt to pull a fast one. Now go and make others aware for they will protect you. At your beck and call, if you should suspect or come upon an infiltrate, it is time to drain the swamp!

At your service to report a scam:

- USA.gov
- Consumer.FTC.gov
- Fraud.org

Remote PC Repair Scams - originated out of India, representatives claim that the consumer's computer is infected and can be fixed with their help. The representative will use this time to infect the computer and force the owner of the computer to make a payment for unnecessary work over the phone by credit card.

Fake/Counterfeit Scam - originated out of China, online stores mimic legitimate companies selling popular items. The goal is to get the consumer to make purchases, get the personal information and then sell it on the black market. If you want to authenticate, then contact the brand name company.

Fraudulent/Fake Check Scam - a consumer receives an elaborate email detailing how they are having trouble cashing a check, whoever responds to the request will receive an added bonus for their trouble. The endorsed check will bounce and the victim will be left with no money.

Pets-for-sale Scam - A fake website offers pet adoptions or asking for a donation. Payment consists of Insurance and shipping fees. Pay by moneygram, western union or a non-returning money transfer to an overseas bank. ScamGuard can assist with securing information of reliable animal breeders in your area.

Grant Scam - Scammers legitimately purchase consumer information from top corporations. Scammers pose as government officials that have a unique opportunity to offer grant money for a processing fee.

Collection Agency Scam - a representative of a fictitious collection agency that threatens a lawsuit unless the consumer settles their debt.

House/Vacation Rental Scam - Scammers advertise fictitious properties for rent, they will only converse with prospective renters via VOIP phone numbers located in a Foreign country. First months payment must be made via a money transfer.

Payday Loan Scam - Scammers focus on the vulnerable consumer. Fake website representatives call consumers and relay that they have qualified for a low interest loan.

Student Loan Scam - A US Department of Education seal does not mean it is legitimate. Deal directly at StudentAid.ed.gov to check on your options for student loan debt.

* If you stop payments to your loan, it will hurt your credit.

Common Scams:

The trickery continues and only the trusting and vulnerable will be taken advantage of. So be wise and make your next move the right one!

- Advance fee scams
- Chain letters
- Charity scams
- Dating scams
- Debt relief scams
- Free security scams
- Government grant scams
- Health product scams
- International financial scams
- IRS-related scams
- Job scams
- Jury duty scams
- Mass Mailing Fraud
- Military romance scams
- Phantom debt scams
- Pyramid schemes
- Scams that use the names of the FBI or CIA
- Service members or veteran scams
- Smishing, vishing and phishing
- Social Security imposter scams
- Subpoena scams
- Tech support scams
- Text message spam[139] [140]

CHAPTER 5

THE VISION OF A REAL LIFE WARRIOR

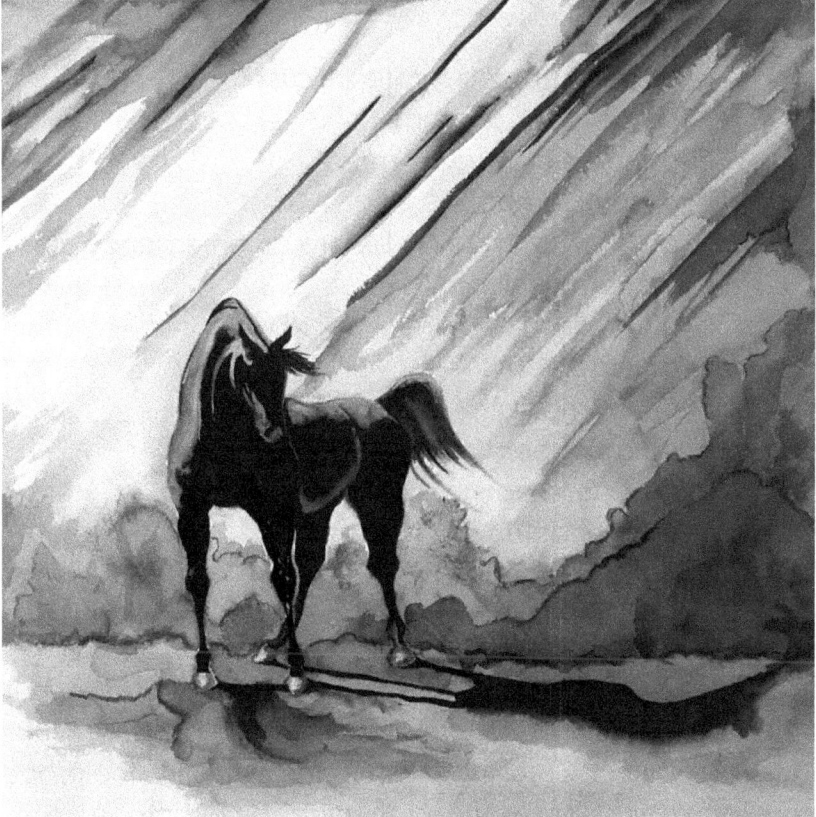

Artist Alisa Chmielinski

Men and women who have built, strengthened, and prepared for what the future has in store, who knows priority is staying one step ahead, strategically planning for the next move.

Everyone does battle, averting crises as they suddenly arise. Maneuvering life's twists and turns, changing careers, maintaining family, and relationships.

- What will you do?
- Will you be prepared for life's tricks?
- Will you be weak or strong?
- Will you settle or strive for more?
- Will you love or hate?
- Will you know what to do before an emergency arises?
- Will you communicate?
- Will you protect?
- Will you compromise?
- Will you tell the truth?
- Will you be respectful?
- Will you extend your hand to others?
- Will you strengthen your foundation?
- Will you win the war?
- Will you be the warrior with the golden heart?

Life's dimensions, the circle of wellness surrounds us all and it is of the utmost importance for our survival. The balance is like a machine with many moving parts. If one part fails, the process breaks down and you will need to be ready to compensate.

Life is a team effort so the Savvy Kid will build a support system, it will be in place waiting, in a time of need.

As I maneuver life knowing and understanding the balance, it is important that I look to see who I have surrounded myself with. I have built a support system of others with integrity, values, morals, ethics, and honesty. Respected for who they

160

are and what they do. They are Warriors, they are Real Life Heroes.

Real Life Heroes make the world go round and so do you. As Warriors do, we will continue to fight together to win life's battles and accomplishments.

Look around you, surround yourself with others who are caring and good, who will support you in times of need.

If you have a problem, find a solution. When you find a solution and become strong, help others. If others do not want help, you yourself must continue to move forward, one step closer to becoming a success, a Real Life Hero.

It is an honor to present those who have walked in my path and are willing to tell you their story, so others may realize that it is real. It can be done, hopes and dreams can and will come true, for we are all in this together.

REAL LIFE HERO ALONZO CEASAR BURNHAM - RETIRED POLICE OFFICER

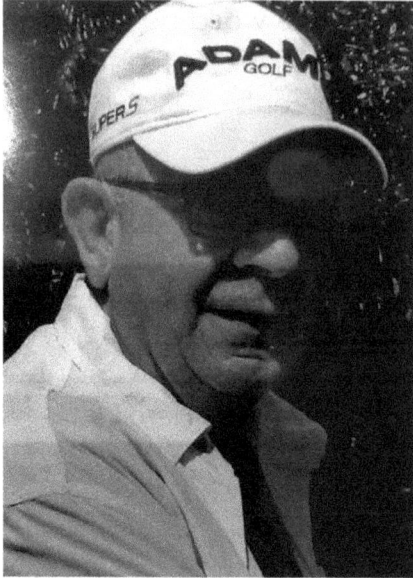

A man of strength and stature. A Protector on and off the job, who put his life on the line everyday he put his uniform on. To me, he is stability, safety, and security, my protector as a child, my world. He is my dad. The man I go to when I have a question, need guidance, but above all, because there is nothing more important than family. The man who stood for and taught me about respect, control, integrity, honor, and truthfulness for starters. He instilled the importance of detail in me at a very young age, something I use on a daily basis.

At age 12, sixth-grader Alonzo made the papers, all because of Roger the dog. Roger followed Alonzo to school and absolutely refused to leave without him. He kept a vigil at the front door, and when the door opened, he ran in, right to him. Roger later developed an even better strategy in his cold war against school authority, no one would keep him apart from his master. If he was shut out of the school, he would climb up the fire escape, outside Alonzo's homeroom. Nott Terrace elementary school finally gave in, and Roger was admitted for a higher education. Roger's presence in the school was a victory. A story of a boy's affection for his dog, and a dog's devotion to his master.

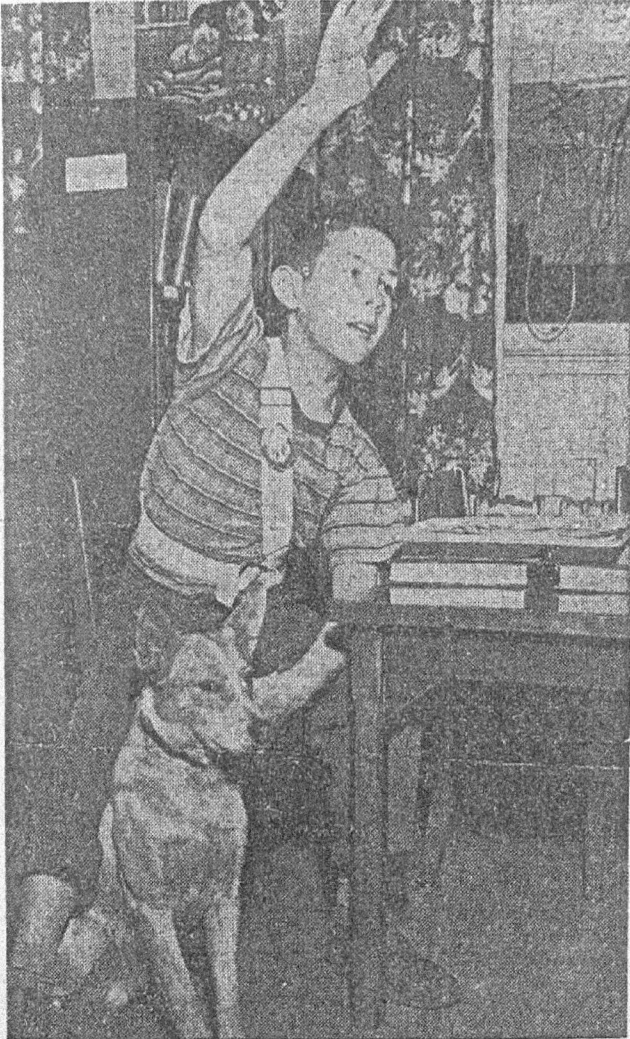

PUP-LIC SCHOOL—Roger, who is Alonzo Burnham's pet dog, is going in for higher education. Refusing to be left out of class, he finally was "admitted" to Nott Terrace elementary school. He lies at Alonzo's feet, studies the class. That's enough studying for him.

If someone had profiled Alonzo at the age of 12, the report would have shown that he showed characteristics of a police officer, and that is what he became. A man of honor. A straight shooter, there was never a question as to what he meant. He was the law, he put his life on the line every day to help serve and protect. Everyone got a fair shake, it didn't matter who you were or where you came from, he always did the right thing.

If you were on the wrong side of the law, watch out, he would track until he caught the prey. He kept the streets of Schenectady, N.Y. clean and safe.

Circulation | SECOND SECTION | SCHENECTADY, N.Y., 12301, MOND.

Delacey Questioned by Police for 11 Hours—
Patrolman Arrests Ex-Convict at Gunpoint

By FRED HOEKSTRA
Gazette Police Reporter

Patrolman Al Burnham, investigating a report of "breaking glass" early yesterday morning at an upper Union street service station, captured at gunpoint a 23-year-old ex-convict currently facing indictment on a felony charge.

JOSEPH DELACEY, 23, of 1554 Foster avenue was questioned for at least 11 hours before breaking down and admitting five burglaries, according to Detective Sergeant John Mullen. He was booked last night on a charge of vagrancy and was being held in city jail without bail.

Deputy Chief Joseph Peters Jr. said Delacey confessed to breaking into Speniard's service station, 1737 Union street early Sunday after first burglarizing Wildau's service station at 1107 Union street where he stole $116.75. The money was found in a Schenectady Trust Co. bag which was in his possession at the time of his capture.

Peters said Delacey also admitted breaking into Wildau's station last month, taking about $25, and breaks at the Boulevard Fruit Garden, 1033 Erie boulevard and at the A&P market in Ballston Spa. A large quantity of cigarets was stolen from the city store while cigarets, radios and watches were taken at the Saratoga county market.

DELACEY'S capture came yesterday about 4:30 a.m. as the result of a woman's call to police headquarters. She told officers she had been awakened by the sound of breaking glass and thought that police lacey a second time — at this point standing in front of a lift about 10 feet away. The officer shouted to Delacey:

"Stand still or I'll shoot."

After a moment's hesitation, Delacey turned and dove under a car which was in the garage for repair.

THE OFFICER didn't enter the station, he explained, because he was alone and didn't know if Delacey had a weapon or if anyone else was with him. One of several other officers dispatched to the scene — Patrolman Thomas Foley — arrived and the officers entered the garage to make the arrest. Delacey surrendered without a struggle.

It was the second time in less than a week that Burnham found himself in a "tough" spot alone and it renewed criticism by other officers regarding the one-man car system. On Jan. 13 Burnham was alone when he walked into the home of a mental patient who is alleged to have stabbed his mother 11 times.

AFTER BEING taken into custody, Delacey was searched and police said they discovered the money bag taken from Wildau's service station earlier.

Brought to headquarters, Delacey was put under intensive questioning by teams of delec-

—(Gazette Photo)

ACCUSED BURGLAR—Twenty-three-year-old Joseph Delacey of 1554 Foster avenue, who admitted five burglaries, is booked at police headquarters last night on a technical charge of vagrancy. Standing to Delacey's right is Patrolman Alonzo Burnham who captured the ex-convict at gunpoint in a Union street service station early yesterday morning. In background is Detective Sergeant Milton Furman. were brought in for questioning. Peters commended the work by youth aid bureau officers of officers involved in yester

Alonzo watched and listened, he observed body language. He could look into your eyes and know if you were telling the truth. He trusted his intuition, and his decision-making skills were unshakable. He was a top cop, welcomed challenges, and fought for what was right. He knew when to give you a break and when to break you. Alonzo kept his friends close and his enemies closer. You wanted him on your side, he did what he said, he was the real thing.

A top athlete, his superior strategic skill came through in his baseball and football career. Making the right moves at the right time, he was a champion. Would you believe me if I told you that he wrestled Victor the bear and pinned him? The truth is he did, and I can prove it.

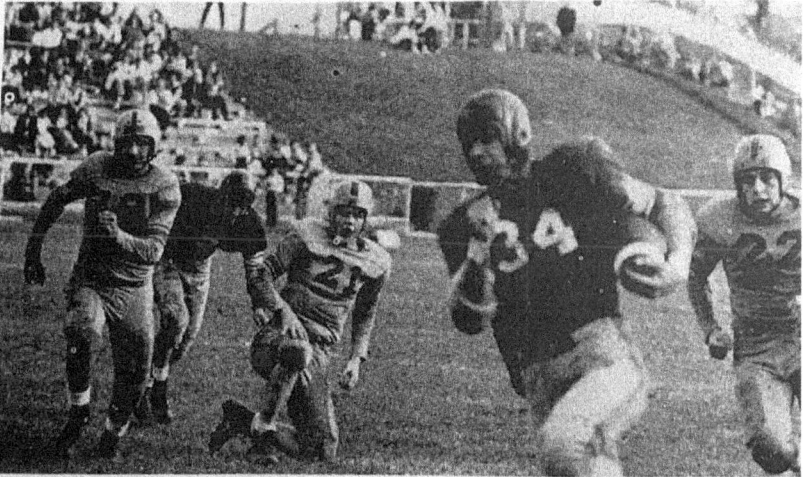

Capital Region Scrapbook: (No) Clash of the titans

They would have talked about the game for decades. Two undefeated Schenectady high school powerhouse

Jeff Wilkin | November 2, 2018

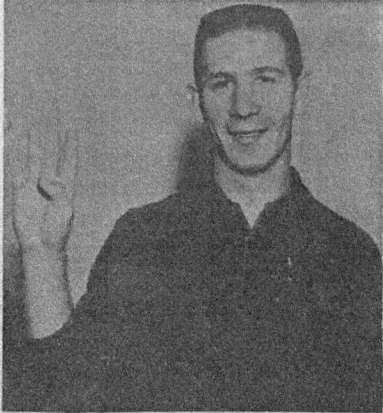

Burnham Had Great Pro Start; Homer on Very First Pitch

No one—but no one—could have started his professional baseball career any more auspiciously than Alonzo Burnham did this year.

The former four-sport ace at Nott Terrace joined Bluefield, W. Va., in the Class D Appalachian League June 25 and hit the very first pitch on his first time at bat for a home run. Whitville, Va., was the site.

"It was a tremendous thrill," says Burnham, back home at 641 Terrace Pl., and awaiting the start of his off-season job as a tabulating machine operator in the State Department Sept. 26.

The 20-year-old, five-footten, 175-pound catcher use that home-run as a warning to Appalachian pitchers. He hit .364 in some 29 games and was promoted to Thomasville, Ga., in a faster "D" league, the Georgia-Florida. He suffered a leg injury in his first game there, went on the disabled list for 16 days and was immediately advanced three classifications to Macon, Ga., in the Class A Sally League.

With its regular catchers, Mike Napoli and Bill Coleman, on the sidelines with injuries, Macon pressed Burnham into immediate service. He caught 11 straight games, went to the bench when Napoli returned for four and caught the last five games of the season. He finished with a .200 average.

Joe Thomas of Albany, area scout for the Brooklyn Dodgers, spotted Burnham playing in the Albany Twilight League early this season and gave him a bonus to join the chain.

Burnham participated in baseball, football, track and wrestling at Nott Terrace. In

ALONZO BURNHAM
... four bases on first pitch!

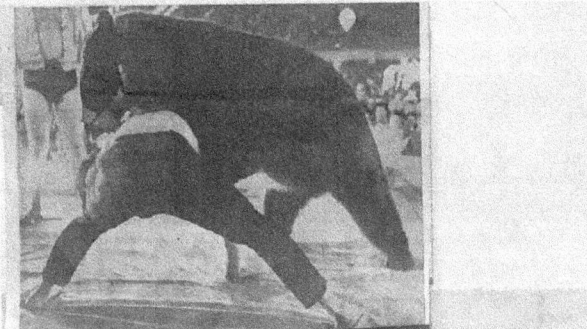

From bear wrestling to crime stopping, he's a top cop

My Dad, My Hero

REAL LIFE HERO BRIAN NEARY - GM AND HOMEOWNER

From Left to Right: Jeff, Delonyx, John, Brian

Handsome, charismatic, and flashes a smile that tells a story. Never underestimate for he is a force to be reckoned with. With a glance into your eyes, he can see your soul and read you like a book. Split-second decisions have paved his way, and he stays true to form. A man of control and unwavering loyalty, nothing is beyond his reach. One day he will take the world by storm if he so chooses.

A modern-day hero. The struggle is real. Enormous responsibility comes with building a new home, constant details must be secured and maintained. Balance and control are tested with long work hours and training to elevate within the workforce. Home life offers both excitement and solitude with the presence of Riley the family dog. She protects her home territory and stands at her master's side, never faltering with her unconditional love. The peaceful support of his soulmate who is loved, cherished, and respected. Life's perfect battle, he has already won the war.

"Let me introduce myself to you. My name is Brian but please call me Bri, all my friends do. Others tell me that they see me as a no-nonsense kind of guy, dry humored, and very well-liked. When looking life in the eye, any challenge that presents itself is gladly accepted with open arms. Maintaining organization and control are two of my specialties. Treating my fellow man like family is my belief in how everyone should be treated.

Strength, motivation, stability, and compassion are a few of the tributes that were handed down to me through my family. My drive and motivation come from within and what will happen when I succeed? I will repay the love and support to my family and friends. Thinking of a strong foundation of morals, values, and ethics, two powerful words come to mind - Honesty and Respect - something that stays with me and is practiced on a daily basis, my mother taught me young. My choice of a "business" career comes from a deep life-long baseline instilled in me—starting with saving change, rolling coins, bank accounts, stocks and bonds, not to forget the early mention of a retirement fund.

The love of life and positive thinking will lead me to succeed, "The way you think is the way you go." It is worth fighting for what you believe in rather than accepting just anything.

My beliefs and hard work brought me to the point in my life where I had my first home built, an addition to my portfolio."

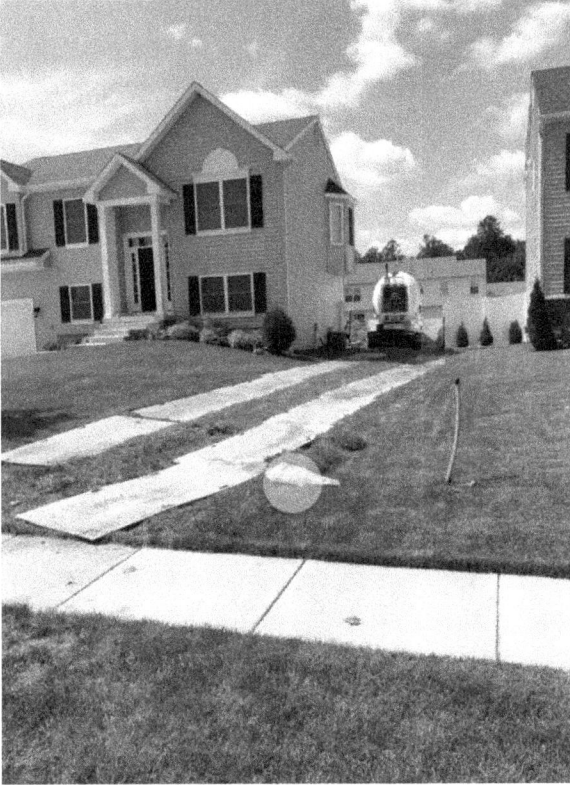

Brian's Tips:

The smartest strategy to have a home built is to go into it with your eyes wide open, know every expense and budget for it. Just to give you a heads up if you plan on going down that path:

Pros:
- Feeling of success
- Investment in your future
- Project management experience
- A home for your family
- Ability to leverage money
- Personal Paradise
- Tweak to your own liking
- Positive credit impact

Cons:

- Potential overwhelming responsibility
- Long-term financial burden - 15 yr vs 30 yr mortgage
- Taxes, taxes, taxes
- Personal liabilities
- Low liquidity (Asset)
- Credit risk if you fail - pre-foreclosure, short sale, bankruptcy

REAL LIFE HERO HELEN KATHRYN - DOCTOR

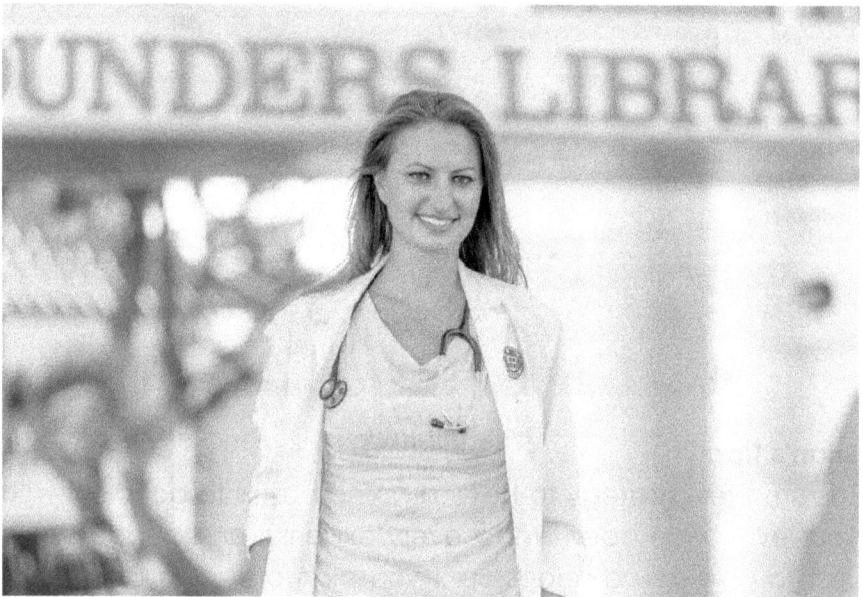

Beautiful and intelligent, she is a lady of all dimensions. Her life is dedicated to the betterment of others. Endless hours of learning and training, at times, to the point of exhaustion. MD will follow her name, and she will stand with the specialists, for she will never give up her fight to protect the ones in need. Her presence is like a beam of light shining down, with a glow that brings a feeling of calmness. A gift to behold.

A modern-day hero. A healer of the sick and empowerment of the well. Half the battle is realizing you are not in this fight alone.

Striving for excellence and accepting nothing less, the mind is intolerable to the thought of defeat. Giving with every ounce of strength, she will find new ways to cure, a caretaker of mankind, home, and self. A peacefulness overcomes her as her soulmate watches over and protects her. Life's perfect battle, as she has already won the war.

"I wanted to be a doctor starting from age five. My road has been anything but straight, I had a lot of trouble with depression during my undergraduate years which torpedoed my freshman year of college. I spent the next three years doing everything I could do to get my GPA up. Every semester, I had advisers telling me to change my end goal of med school by constantly saying "No," and "It's not possible." I knew they were wrong, I felt the calling deep within to keep pushing and find a way. I heard about a Caribbean medical school by chance, and by that point, I had unfortunately started to believe them. So once I graduated from USF with my bachelor's degree in Science, I joined the workforce as a consultant for hospital billing.

"After about six months, I realized I was not ready to give up on trying to become a medical doctor. I secretly applied to Saint George's University in the hopes that I would get an interview, but if it did not work out, I would not have to deal with the pitying looks from my loved ones. Fortunately, I was granted an interview and announced the good news to my family. They were extremely excited and supportive. I was admitted to the MD/MPH dual degree program and moved to Grenada for two and a half years. I suffer from exceedingly terrible test anxiety, so the USMLE licensing exams have proven to be a challenge unmatched by any other in my life.

"There is no obstacle that proves impossible. It may feel that there are hurdles in your life that you feel like you cannot overcome but ignore that thought process. KEEP PUSHING ALWAYS. There is no person that goes through life without strife, the difference is how you meet challenges in your life. There were so many instances where I wanted to quit, throw in the towel, and find some other option that wasn't as hard. But the best things in life, the most important things in life, are the hardest. The most difficult challenges you keep fighting through are the most valuable. I know because I lowered my shoulder and battered through the barriers. If you believe that you are an unstoppable force of nature, you will be.

Being able to give to others in such an important way is such a gift. Being a doctor is so much more than science. It is seeing and being human in the most primal way. When people are sick and/or dying, they need others in a way that is completely different from anything else. And being able to offer the support and human connection they need and want is such a profound experience. I not only get to be a solution, but I also get to be an integral supporting part of the journey. The true treasure of humanity is leaving a positive mark on another person's life, and this career offers that thousands of times over. It is an unmatched experience to work in healthcare."

Helen's Tips:
You have to be passionate. It is the most difficult thing you will ever do in your life. Understand that although it can be all encompassing, do NOT lose sight of your life, be a person that is a doctor/medical student, NOT a doctor/medical student that is a person.

REAL LIFE HERO MARK BURNHAM - BUSINESS OWNER, REALTOR, CONTRACTOR

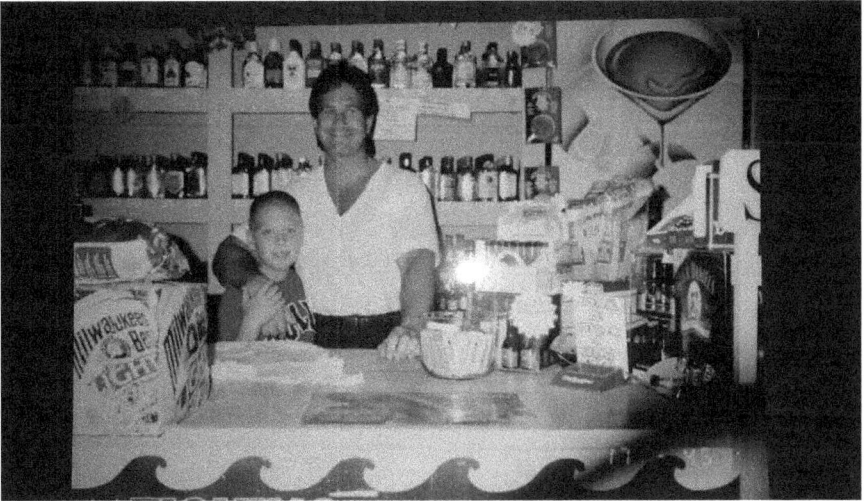

Tall, dark, and handsome with a quick wit. Mark could have easily made a career in the movies. A man who would give you his last dollar and would extend a hand to anyone in need. Partners in crime when we were little, we used to awaken in the early morning hours on Christmas day and sneak out to the living room where Santa had left our presents. An unbreakable sibling bond was formed, and although we are miles apart, memories are forever.

A hero who left home at a young age to pursue his dreams of owning his own business. Mark was successful, building and sculpting with his bare hands, building a home is an art. A store owner has come easy, for he is a friend to all, a warm heart that will never cool. The work takes long hours, laboring, and takes its toll on the joints but will be viewed as a masterpiece. His foundation of morals, ethics, and values are impenetrable. High emotional intelligence and strong in mind, body, and soul, he is loved and respected by all.

"Knowing it was time to branch out and pursue a career, I left the city of Schenectady, New York and traveled south settling in Rehoboth Beach, Delaware.

It was the beginning of being my own boss. Setting goals and expectations according to the highest standards. The mission I lived by was "treat others as I would like to be treated."

Flipping houses, building homes, becoming a realtor and becoming a bar owner were just a few ways to bring in income.

The responsibilities of a businessman begin with providing five-star customer service, listening, and maintaining social connections. It is like playing a chess game and knowing when to make the right move at the right time.

The bar was converted into a package store, which changed the environment of music, games and some hootin' and hollerin' to beverage and grocery.

Building and flipping homes is quite a delightful challenge. The completed project is a work of art and leaves a feeling of accomplishment."

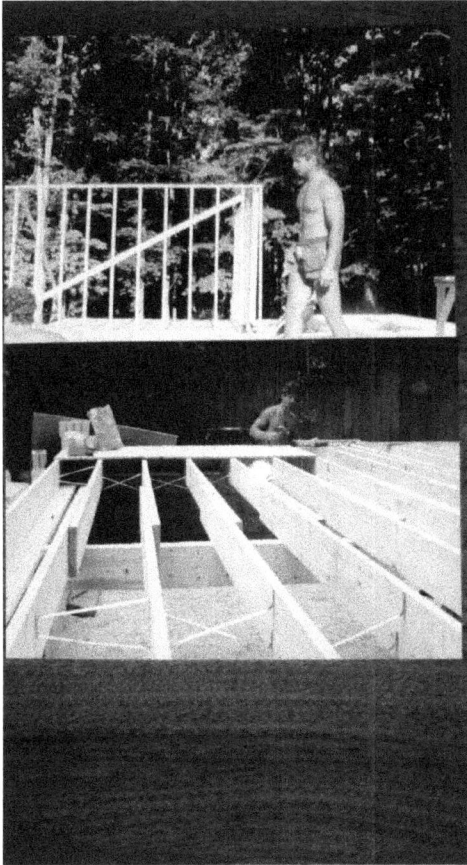

Mark's Tips:

- Hard work.
- Treat others with respect.
- Maintain friendships.
- Read your contracts thoroughly.
- Keep in strong physical shape to prevent injury.
- Maintain cash flow to get projects started with supplies.
- Consider real estate because it will never go away.
- In the alcohol industry - do not be your own best customer.
- Use proper body mechanics when lifting.

REAL LIFE HERO AMANDA CHMIELINSKI - BARTENDER, STUDENT

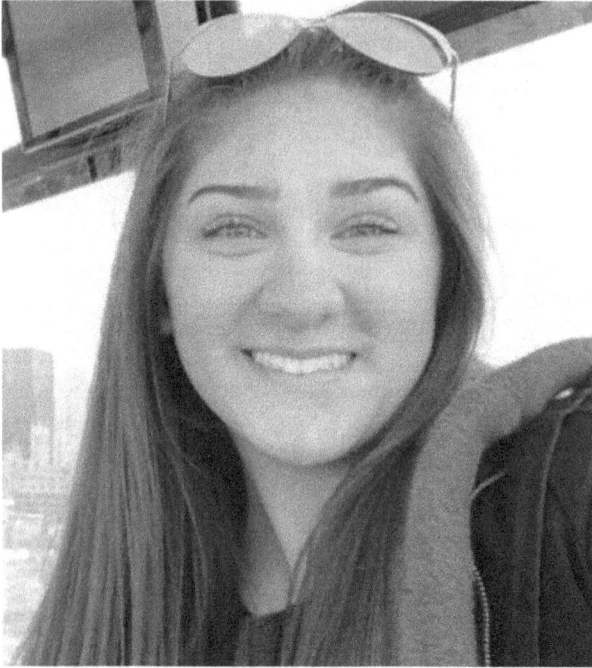

Soft-spoken, reserved, and a smile filled with warmth. The 'art of elegance' would be a better description. An inner strength, so quiet on the surface, propels a forward motivation. Life will be lived to the fullest extent and the expectations will be on a higher level. A character of integrity and untouchable loyalty.

A modern-day hero, stunningly beautiful and intelligent. Amanda has taken the reins of responsibility and possesses the skill of split-second decision-making with maturity beyond her years. A college student, waitress/hostess and friend to all. Her two loyal pets, Bubba and Tabby, wait patiently for her to return home. In pursuit of her dreams, soon they will become a reality, a career woman in the making. She carries the aura of an angel.

"When I was young, I started taking on responsibility, saving my money along the way, keeping instant gratification at bay. I know that the long-term goal takes priority along with extending my education. The plan is to attend a community college at a cheaper rate while I get a few of the liberal arts classes completed. I will then move up to the state college and attain a degree. The bottom line is to think money smart and not develop a large amount of debt before I graduate.

My end goal in mind is to get a degree in Criminology and Forensics. So the challenge is to create a world of balance. Working as a waitress is a temporary job to pay for living expenses and that also includes taking care of my two beautiful cats, Tabby and Bubba. It is an eye-opener, to say the least, when you become responsible for yourself and also the care of animals. I believe it is life's way of preparing us for parenting and it teaches us what will be needed for the job.

Be prepared to be sleep deprived, eat healthy, organize your time, and keep up with your studies. Reach for your hopes and dreams, taking into account that the only one that can stop you is yourself."

Amanda's Tips:
- Stay calm and courteous.
- Customers always come first.
- Be outgoing and social.
- Be empathetic and make others feel comfortable.
- Walk out to the car with a friend or escort after work for safety.
- Dress appropriately.
- Walk away from inappropriate comments.
- Report to your boss if you feel uncomfortable.
- Be a team player at work.

REAL LIFE HERO ALISA CHMIELINSKI - K9 TRAINER/HANDLER, ARTIST, STUDENT

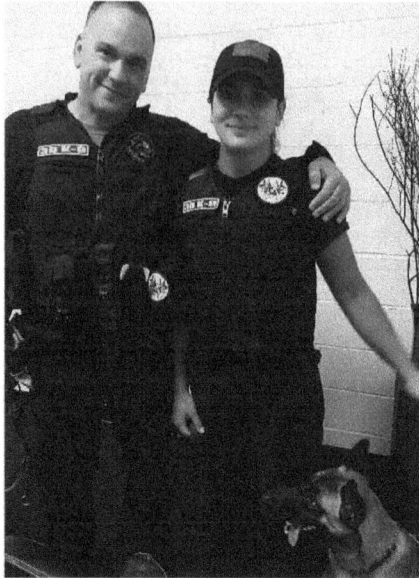

Left: Mark Chmielinski; Right: Alisa Chmielinski

Young, intelligent, and beautiful, her quietness carries a sense of intrigue. Multitasking at its best to say the least, and working seven days a week with not even a hint of complaint. In pursuit of a career, while training and working as a K9 Handler, she is unstoppable.

A hero and a leader. Alisa is saving lives with her team, K-9 Banchi and Wasabi. For every drug that she can confiscate, a life may be extended. She carries an unwavering strength and responsibility. Her talents are endless and will continue. In pursuit of her dreams, a career woman in the making. She will break the glass ceiling barriers with the strength of a breathtaking tigress.

"My main goal is to continue my education as a college student and obtain a degree in Graphic Design, Criminal Justice, K9 Specialist or maybe all three.

"Working while attending college is a priority to succeed. The struggle is real and expenses must be paid. Gas, food, clothes, entertainment, and vehicle repairs just to mention a few.

"The love of the K9 is quite the challenge, it is imperative to gain their trust so that a bond can form. They must know the job that is required of them and follow a command without wavering. I am the master, the handler, and the caretaker, which requires great physical strength and restraint. Caring for the K9 includes bathing, feeding, training, exercising, and up to date medical care for a healthy status.

"This job is not for everyone and you must have a love for animals. Training for narcotic and explosive scent detection is the end goal and extends into the area of re-entry homes, rehabs, residential homes, prisons etc. With a find, comes a great sense of accomplishment but a degree of high risk is involved. One must keep walking, no eye contact and maintain a no-nonsense demeanor, never to break mentally.

College can be mentally exhausting and training canines is physically exhausting. Sleep deprivation soon sets in but in the end, the reward will be great.

Looking into all the possible opportunities life has to offer, the increasing responsibilities have become all too real and the need for strong intuition and decision-making skills is at the forefront."

Alisa's Tips:
- Strive for balance.
- Move forward with a college education.
- Eat healthy.
- Maintain your physical strength.
- Keep your end goal in mind.
- Keep a strong work ethic.

REAL LIFE HERO DAVE BURNHAM - BUSINESS OWNER

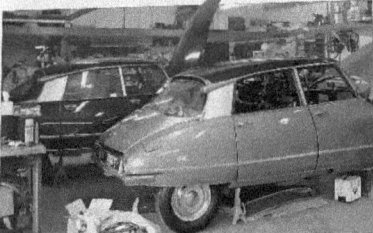

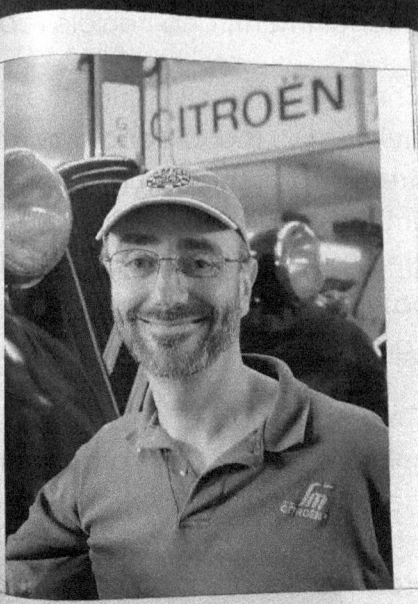

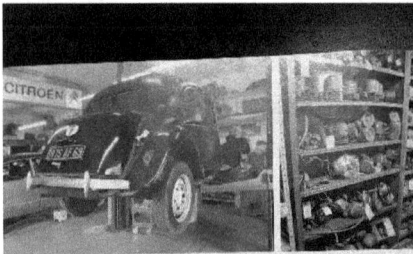

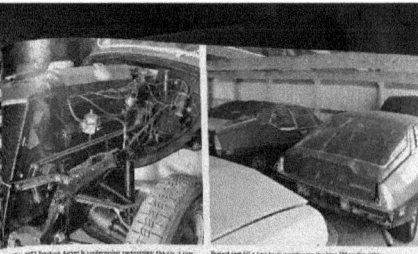

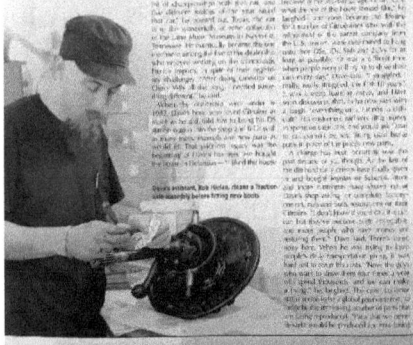

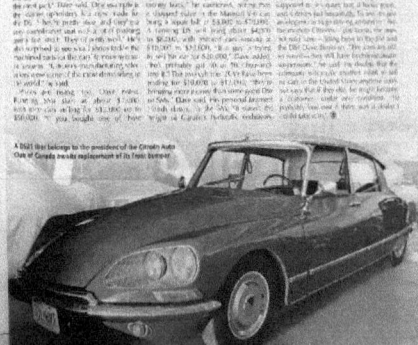

A humble man who will tell you he just got "lucky" in business. The opportunity appeared at his doorstep, but it was his intellect and his go-with-the-flow personality that brought him to the highest level, to be known internationally. It has been an honor to have him for my cousin.

A kind, thoughtful hero. Long hours, hard work, and giving back brought him to leadership in business, cars, and racing. His foundation is strong and he strategically set up a retirement plan early on. Genuine and sincere is who he is and he treats his customers like family and with respect. His reputation precedes his character, for he is genuine, sincere, and listens because he cares.

Daves Tips:
- Above all, be honest.
- Be compassionate of a customer's situation and go the extra mile to help.
- Keep retirement planning at the forefront of your mind. Something as simple as a large garage, building, or warehouse on your own land that would house vehicles during the off season for a monthly charge.

REAL LIFE HERO HAROLD BURNHAM - RETIRED GE

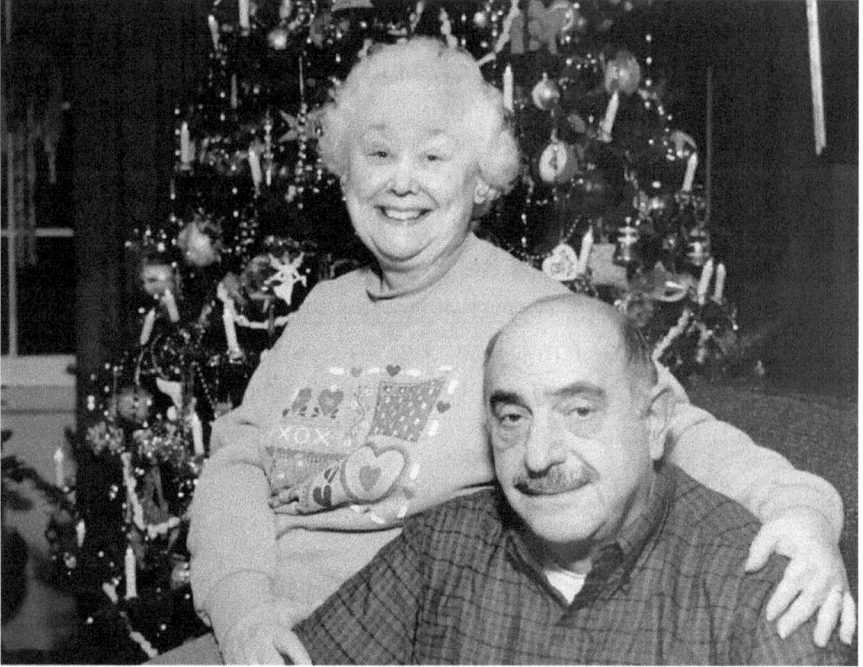

Left: Frances Burnham; Right: Harold Burnham

A man of belief, sincerity, kindness and of genuine action. A prime example of possessing a foundation made of steel, financially secure, and psycho-socially balanced. Charity giving is a priority through sponsorship and brings hope and motivation to others less fortunate, and for that, he will be blessed forever. Aunt Fran has passed but she leaves behind some of her writings about Uncle Harold.

★PREFACE★
★ ★ ★

Now in the sunset of our lives, I felt that it was finally time to deal with the Army life of my husband, Harold Ernest Burnham. We were married on March 2, 1957, and it has taken me all of those fifty years of marriage to obtain the facts for this account. I asked him about it many times over the years, but it seemed still too close to when the events happened to sort it all out, or even for Harold to take those years seriously. There were, however, two words that consistently slipped out and they were "Alaska" and "flood". Writing this account in 2007, I finally finished it in 2008, and in the process found that a lot went on besides Alaska and flood, even if it was not exactly earthshaking.

In 1949, four years after the end of World War II, the U.S. Government discontinued the draft that had been started in 1940. Just a matter of months later, in 1950, after the Korean War broke out, the seriousness of that new conflict reinstated the draft.

The Korean War ended in 1953 about eight months before Harold was drafted, but the Cold War continued. The Cold War started back in 1945, at the end of World War II, and became increasingly tense in the late 1940s and 1950s. It was the reason the draft was necessary, to protect our Country and others from the threat and aggression of Communism.

Although Harold was not called upon to actually fight in a war, he and his fellow servicemen from EVERY branch of service all around the world were trained and ready. In the meantime, they worked and lived the military life and did what they were called upon to do.

Within that military life they also celebrated holidays like Thanksgiving and Christmas. Good for morale, the Army cooked holiday dinners and decorated Christmas trees. Holidays brought back memories and when the soldiers remembered their holidays back home, it helped to put in perspective, at least to some degree, the reason they were in service, which was to protect the American way of life with all of its flaws, treasured so dearly by all.

I always felt that if I could put Harold's Army experiences all together as in the following account, it would not only make an interesting story for our sons, David Harold Burnham and Bryan Harold Burnham, it would also be interesting and important to me.

Before the beginning of the Army account, however, I decided to include a brief history of the little boy who grew up to be a U.S. soldier and what he has accomplished since his Army days. I hope you enjoy reading all of it as much as I enjoyed writing it.

Frances Nellie (Pauley) Burnham
★

- A -

THE ARMY LIFE
and
CHRISTMAS

DRAFTED!

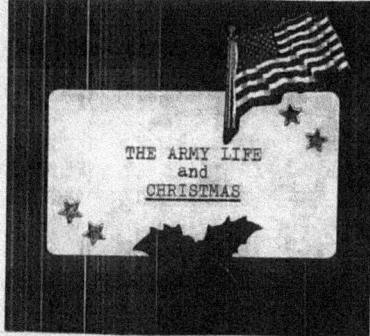

When Harold turned eighteen in 1952, he was going to Nott
Terrace High School in Schenectady, New York. The law at that
time required all young men at the age of eighteen to register
for the draft. The local Selective Service Office was located
over the Central Fire House on Erie Boulevard in Schenectady,
so that is where Harold registered, just like all of the other
eighteen year old locals.

One day in early 1954, Harold arrived home from his job as
a butcher at the Pennywise Market on Nott Terrace, which was
around the corner from his family's home at 641 Terrace Place.
As he opened the door, the first thing he heard was his mother's
voice exclaiming, "YOU HAVE A LETTER FROM THE UNITED STATES
GOVERNMENT!"

The letter came from the Selective Service Office and it was
about to change Harold's life. Like all of the other young men
around the Country about his age, he KNEW that sooner or later
the draft would catch up with him, so the letter was no surprise.

The letter instructed Harold to report to Albany, the State
capital, for an Army physical. After PASSING that physical,

The Vision Of A Real Life Warriors

another letter arrived and THAT was the big one. Dated February
26, 1954, the form letter was sent from local Draft Board #30 and
was a greeting from the President of the United States, who also
is our Country's Commander-in-Chief.

The letter indicated that Harold was Selective Service number
30-30-33-469 and instructed him to report to the local Draft Board
on March 24, 1954, for forwarding to an induction station. On the
appointed day it stated that the local Board would be over at the
Elks Club at 615 State Street in Schenectady, which at that time
was located on the left side of the old Plaza Theater building.
Harold was to bring the form letter and sufficient clothing for
three days, and just in case any local lad decided to IGNORE
the formal directive, the Federal Government included the following
warning:

> "Willful, failure to report promptly to this
> Local Board at the place specified above and
> at the hour and on the day named in this notice
> is a violation of the Selective Service Act of
> 1948, and subjects the violator to fine and
> imprisonment."

The message was clear, but Harold actually looked FORWARD to
ending his butcher job at the family-owned, Pennywise Market. He
had already worked there for a few years and although the Lauricella
family were friends of his and as his employers had been good to him,
as a young, healthy male he wanted to learn new things, make more
money and get on with his life. Before receiving his draft notice,
he had ALREADY applied to the General Electric Company for its
Apprentice Program. Unfortunately there were at least 300 men on the
list before him and it would have taken a year or more to reach the
top of that list, so the United States Army would not be a bad idea
for him at all.

★

Harold's family spread the word through the family grapevine
and to their friends, that he would be leaving for the armed services
soon. Those that could dropped by the house to say goodbye and to
wish him well. Some of them already had family members in a branch
of service. It was a time in history when THOUSANDS of families
across the Country were facing the same separation.

★

When Harold woke up the morning of March 24th, he said his goodbye to his mother and father before they both left for work at the
Army Depot on Westcott Road in Rotterdam. They hugged, kissed and

cautioned him to "BE CAREFUL!", a typical parental response to
sons going into service.

A short time later he also said goodbye to his brother Al, who
would not leave the house until after Harold left. Al was a student
at Nott Lerrace High School, which was only a short distance from
the house.

When Harold walked out of the house that morning he was not sad
about leaving home, it was with a growing sense of adventure. He
said that both he and his hometown buddies just automatically adjusted
to the idea, but that for men who had their careers interrupted,
their response might have been different.

☆

Along with seventeen other draftees from the City of Schenectady,
Harold reported to the Draft Board at 7:30AM on March 24th. They
were given the Mayor's Going-Away Ceremony; an impressive traveling
bag that contained various toiltries from the Mayor's Going-Away
Inductee Committee; a pocket Bible from Gideons International; ciga-
rettes, although Harold did not smoke; coffee and donuts served by
the Salvation Army under the supervision of Senior Captian Clyde
Wadmon; and a chartered civilian bus trip to an induction station in
Albany, New York.

The hosts of the Going-Away Ceremony were members of American
Legion Post 1485 with Jess Huston,Co-Chairman acting as Master-of-
Ceremonies, and George Marzocchi, the other Co-Chairman.

The speakers were Dr. Frank Marra, City Councilman and Acting-
Mayor; Surrogate Judge William W. Campbell; Rabbi Abraham Grossman of
Hamilton Street Synagogue; Rev. John Swartout of Woodlawn Reformed
Church; and Very Rev. John J. Finn of St. John the Evangelist Church
and Harold's own Pastor. It was an inspiring, full and varied
program.

James W. Burch was named Leader of the group of draftees leaving
that Wednesday morning from Draft Board #30, which covered the City
of Schenectady in Schenectady County. Just two days before from
Draft Board #31, which covered Schenectady County OUTSIDE of the City
of Schenectady, fifteen other draftees had also been inducted.

After the conclusion of the Going-Away Ceremony, Harold and the
others, which included some buddies from Harold's high school and
from around his neighborhood, were driven by bus to the Induction
Station in Albany to raise their hands and be formally sworn into
the U. S. Army.

THE ARMY LIFE & CHRISTMAS   Page 4

At the Induction center in Albany, the Schenectady County draftees were joined by more draftees from the City of Albany in Albany
County. When the induction was over, they were all handed box
lunches and put back on buses for the four hour drive to New Jersey.
When the bus pulled out of Albany, Harold knew that his life as he
knew it no longer existed and his life was no longer his own.

****
****

A hero with a forever faith, a serviceman that we thank every
day for our freedom. A family man, caretaker, and protector,
has stood by his faith without exception. His non-judgmental

nature puts you at ease and he will stand by you in the time of need. He believes in helping others and is truly a blessed man.

REAL LIFE HERO JIM DUIGNAN - BUSINESS OWNER

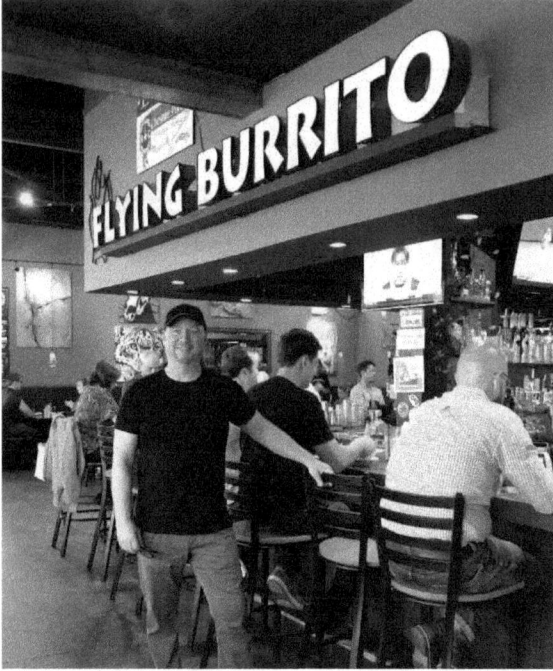

A businessman with style is the first thing that comes to mind. Taking on the corporate world and turning it into something meaningful. The first-hand knowledge of how to treat the customer right and with respect puts his dream in the palms of his hands. A recent addition to the family, he is now a grandpa, a treasure worth far more than all the money in the world.

A real-life hero who has been a tremendous success, an expert at starting up businesses. Customer service is his strength and because he treats his customers like family, his business is flourishing. Long hours, hard work, and a strategic mind brought him to where he is now. A vision of kindness, strength, and stability brings a network of everlasting family and friends.

"I worked long and hard to be where I am today. It started with a degree in Marketing and Management from Siena College in Upstate New York. A training program for managers presented itself, so I went to work for Domino's Pizza, quickly rising to Operations Director and opening my first Dominoes restaurant in the year 1984. Success was real and in 1987, I was awarded the Franny Award from the International Franchise Association, there were only nine winners in the country.

Jim Duignan, pizza king

by Lisa Marie White,
assistant director of public relations

Imagine the following conversation between you and your dad after your Siena Commencement:

Dad: So what are you going to do now?

You: I'm going to work at Domino's pizza

Dad: '@#$?&*!?? !&?$#@'!!

A similar conversation really did take place in 1981 between James M. Duignan '81 and his father, Thomas.

Today, Thomas Duignan feels a lot better than he did that day eight years ago.

Jim Duignan is big, very big, in pizza. Making and selling countless pepperoni and double cheese and advancing steadily in the Domino's managerial ranks "has made me a millionaire," he admits modestly.

"At the beginning, my father wasn't too happy," Duignan recalled. "The family had spent a lot on my education, and here I was working for $3.75 an hour. At that point, my father wanted me to go into banking or advertising, something a little more lucrative.

"If someone would have told me right after I graduated that I would be this successful at this point in my life, I never would have believed them for a minute," said the 30-year-old pizza tycoon.

Duignan, a Schenectady native who now lives in Davidsonville, Md. (near Annapolis), is the owner/manager of 12 Domino's franchises: 11 in Maryland and one outpost at Catholic University in Washington, D.C. A marketing and management major at Siena, he signed on with Domino's Management in Training program in Rome, N.Y., shortly after graduation.

If Domino's guarantees that any pizza ordered will be delivered in half an hour or less, or the pizza is free. To help keep that promise, Duignan had to learn to complete a pizza in less than 90 seconds. As his training progressed that figure was lowered to 60 seconds.

The guarantee Domino's doesn't offer, though, is that management trainees will be given managerial jobs. But with an eye to the future, and with pizza dough under his fingernails if not in his blood, Duignan completed his training in Rome.

He was promoted to a store manager position, and then to a supervisor's position in Syracuse. He moved to Delaware in 1983 where he supervised operations at Domino's stores from Virginia Beach to Syracuse.

According to the Domino's by-laws, a supervisor has to be in that position for at least 18 months before moving up in the hierarchy. The exact day that he completed 18 months as a supervisor, Duignan applied for and was granted a Domino's franchise in Maryland.

"I was keeping an eye on the areas where I supervised, and I pinpointed Maryland because there is a young, mobile population with a lot of disposable income," he said. "Also, people in that area of the country seem to prefer national or regional chains for their fast food, rather than family-owned pizza shops or diners."

As he gained more capital — and business ex-

Duignan applied for and purchased more franchises.

One of the reasons he chose Domino's back in 1981 was because of its status as an up-and-coming chain with good opportunities for expansion and advancement. Eight years ago, the chain owned 500 franchises; today it owns more than 5,000.

According to BusinessWeek magazine, a low buying price for a franchise was one reason for the boom. In the mid-80s, a franchise could be purchased for $85,000-$130,000, compared to $425,000 for a McDonald's, or as much as $1 million for a Wendy's.

Unfortunately, the boom for Domino's means that most of the lucrative spots for franchises have already been taken.

"We're past the frontier stage in the business," said Duignan. "All the good franchises have been gobbled right up, so right now Domino's is concentrating on pinpointing some of their stores which aren't as successful and pulling them into shape."

Pulling a store into shape is something Duignan is well-versed in. His Hyattsville store, the first of his franchises, has been the highest-grossing franchise in the entire chain for two of the last three years, selling approximately 200,000 pizzas and grossing more than $1.6 million a year. His efforts earned him a 1987 Franny Award from the International Franchise Association. He was one of only nine winners in the country.

In addition to hard work and good business sense, Jim also credits his wife, Sharon, with his success. The two met when they were both manager trainees, and Sharon owned three of her own franchises before they were married.

"She was an excellent supervisor in her own right, and she's a good consultant for me now," Duignan said of his wife, who is now a full-time homemaker. "When I come home from work and I have concerns or questions, she's able to help me out and provide suggestions."

Duignan typically works 10- to 12-hour days, four or five days a week. He goes to his office around 10 a.m. to "check out a few things," and then may meet with a vice president or two to discuss accounting and marketing.

"I also have a lot of one-on-one meetings with store managers, and I also drive around visiting individual stores, sometimes until 8 or 10 at night."

When Duignan gives a lecture to a college or business group, which he often does, he encourages his listeners to stick with one company and work very hard to be successful.

"You really have to be willing to put in the hours if you want to get somewhere," he said. "My other piece of advice is to think about what you want to be versus what you want to have. When I get up in the morning and go to work I think about selling pizza and beating the competition. I don't think about buying a new car."

Duignan is proud of his Siena diploma and said his College experience has given him an extra shot of confidence.

"Getting my degree from Siena has really built up my self-esteem," he said. "The College has a great reputation for its Business Division, and when you show people your resume with 'Siena' on it, their eyes get big." Like a large Domino's pizza?

I am the present owner of the original "Flying Burrito" in Raleigh, NC. The local neighborhood place where memories are made especially with families. Serving kids and being a part of their lives is a reward that will never be forgotten."

Jim's Tips:

The restaurant business requires experience, skill, focus, and a can-do attitude. Be prepared to work all aspects:

- Business
- Marketing
- Management
- Training
- Accounting
- Repair and maintenance

REAL LIFE HEROES BOB & SHERI DUIGNAN

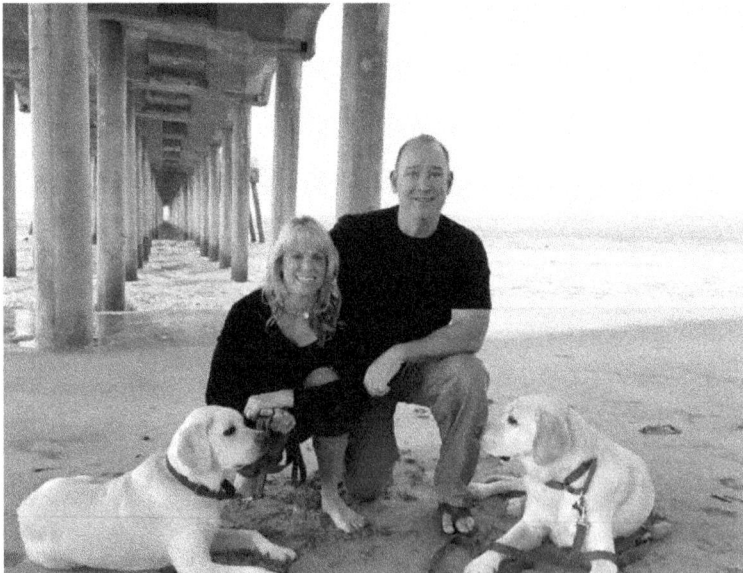

Photography by Jennifer Stroman

The unstoppable duo. Living as one but working separately. That is what comes to mind when I think about this wonderful loving couple. Together, living out their dreams and supporting each other through thick and thin. The dogs look to Bob and Sheri for guidance, caretaking and safety, just as a child would. Parenting skills became a priority and this skillset has been executed with precision. In return, they receive unconditional love from Harley and Auggie.

Each a hero in their own way. A love forever, they will grow old together. They both work tremendously long, hard hours and sometimes are separated due to the jobs. The love, trust, and caring keep them strong when apart and support the dreams of each other. They are well-balanced with friends, family and work. They have met and continue to strive for a successful lifestyle. New and exciting endeavors create change, and they continue to grow together. Loving, kind, empowering and an example of what to do right. They are the picture of success.

Bob Duignan - Senior District Manager

"I work for Fitness International LLC, and City Sports Clubs. I oversee operations at the CSC and LA Fitness clubs, Member Retention Department. Cleanliness, member services, kids club, front desk, vendor relationships and club condition are all priority. Fourteen years of service has brought me in my career to managing 17 clubs, and two district managers that I mentor.

The most rewarding part of the job is working with young adults on their management as well as leadership skills. Many of the district managers have come from within and I am proud to say that I have made a large, positive impact on many.

The travel required for this job means time away from my beautiful wife Sheri, the light of my life. Routines are of great importance to keep things focused and flowing in a positive direction such as lifting weights, cycling classes, and playing flag football. (Not too bad for a 55yr old, right?)"

Bob's Tips And What We Would Look For In This Business:
- People of interest have played team sports, or have been part of a group
- Team, Group, or Activities Captain or President
- Work hard to be part of the above
- Behold passion for fitness

Sheri Duignan - Business Owner

"The proud owner of a franchise in Orange County, CA. I buy houses direct from sellers in tough situations, then fix them up and resell to a new homeowner.

I worked 19.5 years for LA Fitness as District Manager and Vice President. Tired of the corporate stress and learning of HomeVestors simultaneously, it was time to send in the corporate resignation and buy a franchise. Always fascinated by real estate, it led me to buying rental properties for positive cash flow.

I love what I do! Working with the homeowners and being able to help them in a time of need is very rewarding. Improving neighborhoods, seeing the transition fork from being the worst-looking house on the block to the best, is a fun accomplishment.

The job can have some questionables such as fleas, bugs, or other "yucky" unmentionables and sometimes the smells require a mask.

The business is competitive now that HGTV has glamorized flipping houses, but it is a lot of fun when you find one that you can buy."

Sheri's Tips:
1. Stay focused and committed.

2. Persistence pays off.
3. The commitment is huge, both mentally and financially, but, if you put the energy and your heart into it, then it will be well worth it.
4. Get a Coach/mentor. They will help you make fewer mistakes and help you recover from the ones you make.
5. Surround yourself with others in the business.

REAL LIFE HERO KEITH GILLESPIE - REMODELING CONTRACTOR

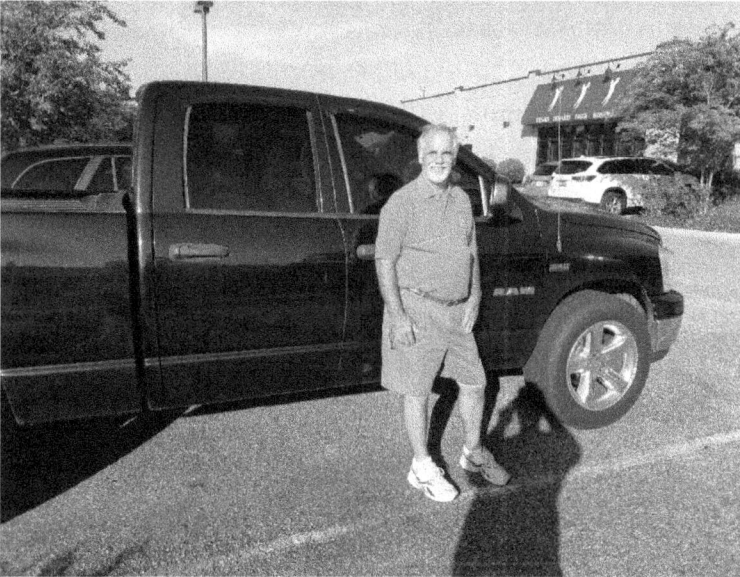

A man with a smile that will melt your heart, laughter that will comfort your soul, and an untouchable stabilizing demeanor. A workforce perfectionist that can take on any home improvement challenge and succeed, as witnessed by many.

A modern-day hero. Keith has been a successful businessman since a young age. His work ethic, attention to detail, and workmanship has brought him success. He learned early on that a balance between work and stress reduction would need to be maintained. Golf was the perfect compensator and that he was superb at. A strong caretaker and protector, he possesses a gift of strength and stability. He is a light at the end of a tunnel.

"I started my business, Keith A. Gillespie Home Improvements, because I have always loved working with my hands. I was never a behind-a-desk type of person. I was interested in woodworking ever since I was a boy. As a young boy in Arizona, I was always watching workers doing construction projects. One year, we had an addition put on the back of the house, and I was more interested in watching the progress than going to school. I would come home right after school and park myself in a place where I could watch what was going on. As the project progressed I made myself available in such a way, that the painting contractor finally asked for my help, in painting the closets.

When we moved to New York, I took shop courses in grade school and high school. The projects that most students made were items such as trinket boxes, chess boards, and cutting boards etc. I made a workbench which had to be transported home with a truck. While in high school during my junior year, I refinished an entire basement for a neighbor down the street, with the exception of the floor covering.

I started to work professionally under a gentleman from Ireland. He was a fantastic finish carpenter and I learned a lot about the field for the next eight years.

After those eight years, I went out on my own and opened Keith A. Gillespie Home Improvements. It was hard work at the beginning, working during the day then going out for estimates at night and on weekends.

As the business grew, word of mouth started to generate more and more work for me. It is very rewarding to see a project go from design to construction and then to finish.

As a remodeling contractor, there are a lot of ups and downs. When you first meet a potential client, you have to be able to sell yourself to them. A good way to do this is to listen carefully to what their desires are. There are always questions about time, quality of work and timing. Most importantly, be honest with the client and yourself. If the project looks too big for you to handle, be honest with them. Tell them what you can actually do for them. If you are always honest and do the best job you can, you and the client will be happy. A happy client means extra work and referrals.

Being in business is not always bright and sunny. There are pitfalls along the way. Money flow can be good and bad at the same time. If there are employees involved it gets even harder. You are running around generating work to keep them busy. As employees help production during the week, no employees means no progress during the week. It is a vicious cycle. That means vacation time may not be in the cards. If you are an honest person and do quality work, this should result in referrals which will help in time off and work for employees. If you use subcontractors for some of your work, this will also help in vacation time.

If a person wants to get into the construction field and does not mind working hard, it is a very rewarding field. Apprenticing under a quality teacher, as well as taking classes at a local vocational school that include construction education and business will help in organizing your business."

Keith's Tip Corner:

Buying a home pre-inspection:
- Check foundation for stress cracks (hairline cracks).
- Look at shingles for sign of cupping (ie. edges cup upward or downward, a sign new shingles needed).
- Check what type of electrical service-breakers or fuses are present (fuses are old style and should be replaced. Costs vary depending on size of new box).
- Septic system or city sewer?
- Well or city water?
- Look at the label on major mechanicals for the serial number (ie. furnace, air conditioning, water heater).
- Look on the internet to find where and when the product was built.
- Look for corrosion on pipes and under sinks at the joints (check water supply for low flow and leaks).
- How old are the appliances? (Newer appliances may need to be replaced in 5 to 7 years.)
- Condition of floors, wood, carpet and linoleum.
- Condition of painting and doors and windows.
- Look under sinks for leaks, flush toilets.
- Run water in drains to check flow.
- Look for mold in the house specifically, at floor baseboard and in the basement.

REAL LIFE HERO MIKE EUSTACE - LEAD TECHNICIAN ENDOSCOPY

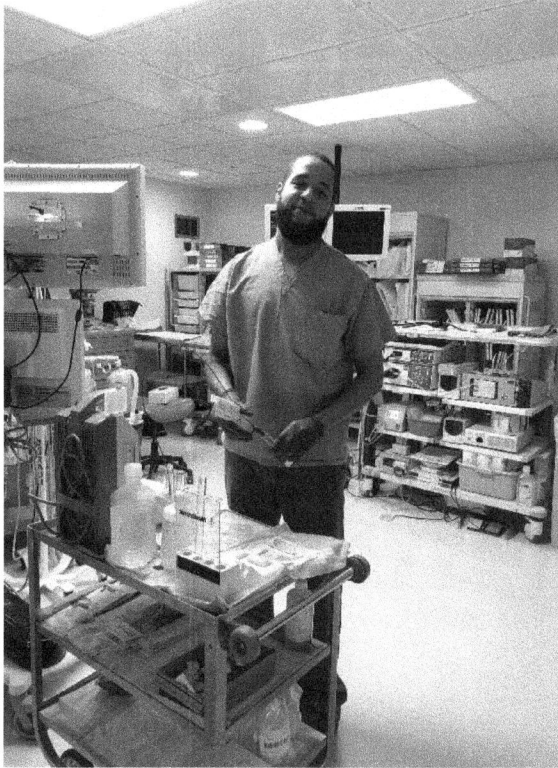

A man with a spirit that will carry him in times of question and certainty. Young, intelligent and respectful as well as respected. His work ethic is untouchable and his caring nature, quick wit, and smile comfort others during times of anxiousness. He will rise to his dreams because he believes in himself, and he will extend his hand and pull others up with him because he is true to heart. One day he will conquer his own interests with a never ending success.

A young modern-day hero. Mike possesses a gift, an aura that he carries when you are in his presence. Mike carries a strong foundation, a strong work ethic, morals, and values. He maintains a wellness balance of work and health. The strategic thinker that he is, he will reach for his dreams and it will bring him the success that he truly deserves.

"My career path started when I worked for five years in a day program for the mentally and physically disabled. The goal was to help the clients be independent and become a part of the community.

I worked in a hospital setting, a fast-paced emergency room, where I learned of a specialty known as Endoscopy. This position spiked my interest and the procedures help others get well and sometimes save lives. In most cases, colon cancer is preventable, and that is why I am here, to keep you out of trouble. I am now "Lead Endo Tech" and will continue to serve.

It is an honor to serve the public and the rewards obtained from helping others is priceless. I am an advocate for the less fortunate and have learned the ultimate truth that those with disabilities have the same needs and wants as others."

Mike's Tips:
- Working in the eye of the public requires continuous learning from both the professionals and the clients. Learning to care for others requires accepting cultural diversity. My belief is everyone I come in contact with is to be treated like I would like to be treated, with respect.

- Education is a priority when working with the public, and I strive to be my best for you. I listen and care deeply about each of you because one day I may find myself in your position.

REAL LIFE HERO JANICE KEENAN - OPERATING ROOM RN, AND GRANDPARENT

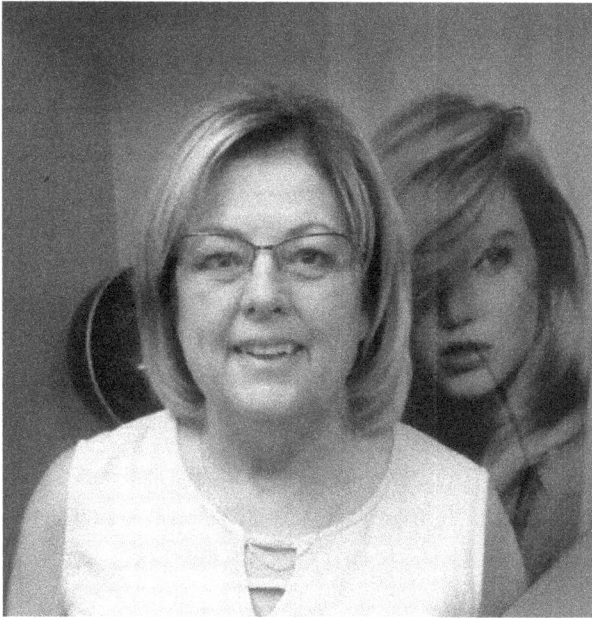

Fast on her feet, quick thinking, and can save your life with split-second decision-making skills. Janice is filled with compassion and lives every day by that code. She is a true nurse at heart, and she is the one you want at your side when you are in crisis.

A true hero at heart. When called in the night for an emergency, there are no questions asked. Janice gives her heart and soul for the sick and treats others as family. With years of experience, she can save your life with her eyes closed. She can hear each breath you take and the pounding of your heart. She runs a tight ship in the operating room, with her, you are in blessed hands. Soon to be a grandma, a reward for all the years of caring for others.

"My career in nursing started in 1981. I followed in my mother's footsteps. After working as a floor nurse both as an LPN, then as an RN, I joined the operating room in 1987. I enjoyed floor nursing very much. I started as a LPN in 1979. I worked on the 3-11 in a small community hospital. Once I graduated as a RN in 1981, I moved to a large hospital in Summit, NJ. Here I worked on the step-down unit to both Medical and Surgical ICU's. This is where my interest in the operating room started. The patients on this floor were very interesting. I enjoyed post-op teaching and helping both the patients and their families.

"After moving to a different part of New Jersey, I was given the opportunity to join the OR staff. This is where I found my calling as OR nurse. Assisting the surgeon in preparing the OR suite, gathering the instruments and supplies needed for each procedure, having the knowledge and experience so that these cases go smoothly. Knowing the surgeon's preferences, the different surgical specialties is always a challenge. Surgical instrument and sponge counts must always be correct in each and every surgical procedure. Focus and precision are utmost for a surgical team, that team works together to make the entire process happen. The surgical team, which involves, the RN, surgical tech, anesthesia personnel, and last but not least the surgeon work together each and every case. When a crisis does occur, we work together for this not to happen, however, if and when they do, the team converges to listen to both surgeon and anesthesia and solve the issue with multiple talents and knowledge working as one.

"I have enjoyed my career as an operating room nurse for the last 30 years. I like to think as myself being multi-specialty OR nurse. My main speciality is general surgery. New and advanced technologies are being developed. Robotic-assisted surgical procedures are the newest in today's operating room.

"The greatest joy is on the way, my son and daughter-in-law are expecting, and I am going to become a grandmother. Parenting skills will come into play but from the viewpoint of a grandparent, the enjoyment factor skyrockets tenfold."

Janice's Tips:

1. I will tell you that one year of Med-Surg is recommended but, one year of ER or ICU nursing will teach split-decision making abilities: how to prioritize, multitask, and learn critical thinking skills.
2. Continued education is important, however, hands-on experience is crucial!
3. Obtain a certification in your specific area such as Operating Room.
4. Maintain your American Heart Association Basic Life Support and Advanced Cardiovascular Life Support (BLS & ACLS) certifications.

REAL LIFE HERO KRISTINA RIJO - REGISTERED NURSE

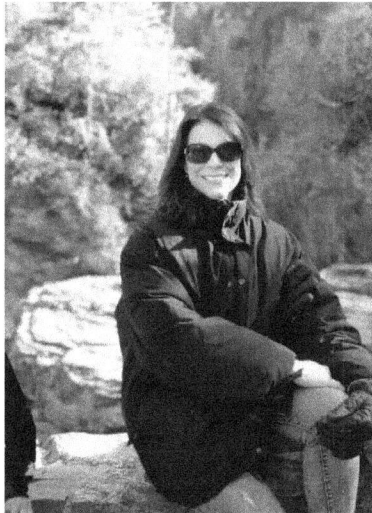

A working single mom, attending school and holding down the fort. She is more like Superwoman. Caring for sick relatives, she wears her heart on her sleeve. Supportive of the kids, she travels the states watching her superstar daughter Courtney play volleyball, breaking all barriers.

A superhero comes to mind. Beautiful, intelligent and an energy that is unstoppable. When life throws Kristina a curveball, she has a gift of turning lemons into lemonade. When she falls, she rises again only higher. A superb parent, she is raising savvy kids. Someday she will look back and ask herself, how did I do it all?

"My career now is a registered nurse, however, I am in school to obtain my APRN certification. I have always loved medicine. Even as a child I had a love for medicine. When my grandmother got sick and passed away, I made the decision to go into nursing so that I could help people and learn more about the disease process. I love what I do and I have learned more about that aspect of nursing than I ever imagined. I really enjoy helping those in need and trying to piece together their symptoms to form a diagnosis. This is something I find myself doing in my everyday life, trying to figure out what is going on with a person.

"What can I say about being a single parent......it is TOUGH!! It is not what I would have chosen for my kids, but this is just the way it was and the way it is. When I was young, I struggled. I made the decision when I was 24 to apply to nursing school.

"I was accepted for the Fall session in 1998 and I started in nursing school in August of 1998, almost 8 months pregnant. I was still married at the time. I delivered a healthy baby girl on October 7, 1998. I missed two days of school and as soon as I was discharged I was back in class. No rest for the weary!

"I was working full time, breastfeeding, married and in nursing school all at the same time. Talk about burning the candle at both ends. I remember sitting in the bathroom pumping my breast during clinicals thinking there is NO WAY I can do this! I did my clinicals on the weekends and attended class twice a week at night. My last semester of nursing school, I switched to weekend days for class and clinicals. I still worked, but only part-time.

"It was in October, one week before my daughter's first birthday, that she got sick. She ended up in the hospital with a septic knee! She was in the hospital for one week and then came home with a PICC line to have antibiotics administered every 6 hours for 6 weeks. While she was in the hospital, I only left one time and that was to take my final exam for nursing school.......and I made an A. I was finally done with nursing school!!

"In 2002, I had another son and in 2012, I had a second son. Courtney was active in cheerleading up until 6th grade and then she transitioned to volleyball. My older son, Christian started playing baseball at the age of 3, and still plays to this day.

"I had a pretty big back surgery in December 2015. During that time, my mom was my caretaker, helping me with my kids and helping my recovery. This was the toughest recovery that I have ever had.

"On October 28, I had to call rescue as my mom was having difficulty breathing. I knew that this was not just the ALS. Once all the testing was complete, it was discovered that my mom had bilateral pulmonary embolism in both lungs and main stem bronchus. After a week in ICU, she was transferred to inpatient hospice to get her pain under control.

"My mom passed away at 12:22 on Christmas day. There are so many things that I wish I had said to her, but instead, I was focused on being strong for her and for my kids. Take it from me, being strong is not always the best road to take, so I will keep her alive in our talks and with pictures.

"Flash forward to 2018, Courtney is a sophomore in college at Francis Marion University. She is playing volleyball and she is killing it!! She absolutely loves it! And yes, I drive up to see her and watch the games typically every other weekend, carefully planning around baseball games. Christian is 16 and is a junior in high school where he plays baseball. Adrian is 6 and he plays multiple sports!!

"Visiting the top of Grandfather mountain, my brother and I spread mom's ashes, at her request. Within one minute of doing so, a huge hawk would fly by, then sat down in front of us. He stayed around 45 seconds and flew off, Mom's way of saying she was ok."

Pros:
You will experience happiness helping people, learning, and expanding my knowledge about nursing and medicine in general.

Cons:
In the beginning, you will work the night shift! Night shift is not bad, however, you will know it is time for a change when you can't remember stopping at a particular stop sign or a light or even remembering driving home! That will scare the hell out of you! Also, everyone including family is always asking you what is going on with this person or that person. I love being a nurse, but sometimes I just want to be Kristina.

Kristina's Tips:
"I can give this if you choose this career when you graduate nursing school go into either ICU or ER, DO NOT GO TO A MED/SURG FLOOR like everyone will tell you to do. I learned

more in the first 6 months working the ER after graduating than I did in nursing school."

REAL LIFE HERO DONNA CLIFFORD - RN, CERTIFIED REGISTERED POLARITY PRACTITIONER

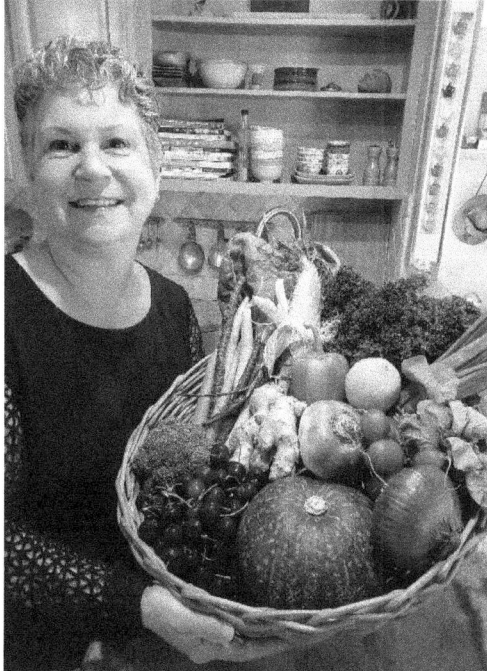

Intrigue and an aura of mastery. She is precise and knowledgeable to the point that she pulls you into her world of macrobiotics. Her art of medicine goes beyond what the conservative alternatives offer. Helping others succeed in their lives and ailments, you cannot put a price tag on. An angel in disguise.

A real-life hero. Donna holds in her hands a realm of medicine that many have overlooked. A healer for the wary that have exhausted their attempts to feel better or be cured of their illness. She maintains, stabilizes, and empowers those that are weak, so they may once again enjoy life. The vision of hopes and dreams, she is a leader in her field.

"Donna Clifford R.N., B.S.N. has thirty-six years of clinical nursing experience, working in the fields of Cardiology, Critical care, and Endoscopy. Specializing in endoscopy, Donna sees the diseases from the inside.

"Donna is also certified and licensed in Massage Therapy and is a Registered Polarity Practitioner. She holds certifications in Body Centered Meditation, Transformational Breathwork, Lastone Therapy, and Chakra Healing. A level four graduate of the Kushi Institute and Planetary Health, she offers consultations and a variety of classes. She owned and operated New Aura, an energetic healing venue incorporating bodywork, meditation, and diet. She has now established an online site for her work. Visit her at Advisemyhealth.com

"If you are faced with a health challenge or want to learn more about living a macrobiotic life, Donna is available for consultation, macrobiotic guidance, cooking classes, lectures, facial diagnosis, and distance healing. Follow her on Instagram and Facebook at Advisemyhealth.

"The point of all this is that macrobiotics is the path back to natural living in a modern world. Preparing whole foods with simple ingredients to balance your child's stress of everyday life cleanses and regenerates his/her mind and body laying down a beautiful foundation for a happy life."

REAL LIFE HERO ELSIE KERNS - SPEAKER, AUTHOR, TEACHER, STRESS SPECIALIST, ADVANCED PRACTITIONER (EDEN ENERGY MEDICINE)

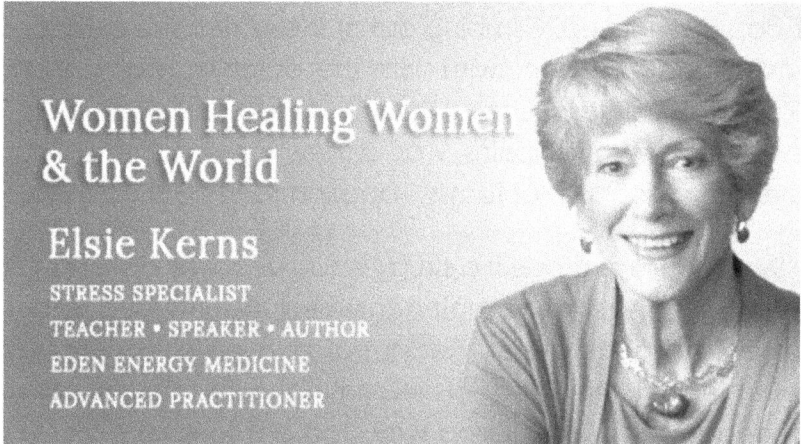

A beautiful, intellectual, kind, gracious, and humorous young woman. When you meet Elsie, the spark in her eyes catches your interest. Established and well known, she steers you down a well-paved path of caring for others. Respect is what follows, her teachings are changing the world.

A hero to all. Elsie is the picture of what an entrepreneur truly is. She has studied under and with the best of her field. Her aura is one of calm and healing. A friend forever, she is strong and dedicated, her focus is unwavering. Blessed with a long reach, she will help many. A vision of beauty, elegance, sincerity, integrity, and honesty, she is not someone you will ever forget.

"People have always been curious about how I went from housewife to healer! It all began swimming with the dolphins during a family vacation in the Florida Keys. Something magical happened.

"Watching the first snowfall dust the earth with a pure white blanket, I started to turn off *Good Morning America* when I was captivated by the contrast of the dolphins spinning the trainer around the water on their fins, then jumping through the hula hoop she held up. Climbing out of the water, she extended the invitation. "You can swim with the dolphins. Call the Dolphin Research Center in Grassy Keys, Florida for details now." In 1987, swimming with dolphins was a new concept and sounded perfect for our Easter family vacation to the Florida Keys!

"Sweaty palms made it a struggle to pull on my bathing suit and one whiff under my armpit confirmed that my deodorant had failed. An accelerated heartbeat and rising anxiety had me questioning this idea of swimming with the dolphins. My teenage sons were asking why Dad got to take pictures while we were being observed by the other guests sitting in the bleachers. The trainer rounded up the ten of us and everyone slipped into the water to meet the dolphins. I floated on top of the water trying to remain calm. I could hear the sonar sounds of the dolphins beneath me as they circled gently around me. They seemed to be trying to assure me I could relax and I did.

"Looking up, I saw my sons whirling around on the dolphin fins, holding the hula hoops and swimming beside several of the dolphins. We were all lost in the magic of the dolphin energy. At the end of the swim, the trainer blew her whistle and called us back to the floating dock. While waiting my turn to climb up the ladder, one of the dolphins suddenly popped up from the under the dock staring at me. The trainer leaned over and whispered, "He wants you to kiss him on his bottleneck nose – go ahead!" Both reluctant and curious, I reached over and planted that first kiss on his nose. The dolphin disappeared under the water and just as I was ready to breathe a sigh of relief, he popped back up looking at me. Okay, a second kiss and then a third. Finally, my turn came to climb the ladder to the dock. The pictures were a wonderful visual revisit of the swim. This past Easter, my younger son, and his wife took their sons to swim with the dolphins at the same research center.

"Something magical had occurred during the swim. I had taken a risk, calmed my fears and felt more open and curious. This curiosity led me to the RAM III metaphysical bookstore in Medford. I didn't even know what the word "metaphysical" meant or why they were using the term "New Age." I just knew that I had to go there. Books on Native American tradition, channeling, meditation, psychic surgeons, healing and more beckoned. Stacked high next to my bed, I began devouring these new concepts around energy and spirituality. Having grown up Catholic, I struggled with the difference between spirituality and religion. Catholicism has a strong structure and definitive ideas while spirituality encouraged me to explore my connection to the divine within me. Learning meditation opened a quiet space internally I never knew was there. Subtle shifts were happening and I knew it all began with the dolphins and those kisses at the dock.

"I began delving into the concepts of spirituality versus my original Roman Catholic upbringing.

"Then I met Barbara Brennan, former NASA astrophysicist and author of Hands of Light, which detailed healing the human energy field. Her 4-year training immersed me in the world of "energy." Additional studies with meditation and Mindfulness-Based Stress Reduction created by Jon Kabat- Zinn encouraged personal introspection.

"Finally, meeting Donna Eden, author of the best-selling book, *Energy Medicine* taught me self-care exercises and healing practices that I could teach others and use myself for maintaining balance, restoring vitality and navigating life successfully. The best part is that everyone can learn and have access to these practical applications 24/7!

"Along the way, I discovered my deep passion for teaching complementary/alternative healing and witnessed the benefits with daily and consistent practice. Anxiety issues I struggled with over the years became manageable and understandable from past experiences. Recurring sinus problems stopped, a healthier diet made a huge difference as did Yoga and Tai Chi for relaxation.

"Now, you might be wondering, what is "energy medicine?" Everything from massage to acupuncture, healing touch, Reiki, Shiatsu, herbal medicine, osteopathy and more fall under the category of energy medicine. In energy medicine, energy is the patient and energy is the healer. In fact, our medical system uses energy medicine with MRI (magnetic resonance imaging), CAT and PET scans. They help reach deeper levels of the human body for diagnosis and work because we are "electromagnetic."

"How do you want to live the next 50 years? The potential to live longer continues to increase. Certainly you want to be healthy and of sound mind. However, the stress response has become the daily norm today leading to chronic illness and autoimmune disorders. Living longer today is a challenge in maintaining vital health, strength, purpose, peace and joy.

"If you would like to explore holistic healing practices, you can begin with meditation, Yoga, Massage, Reflexology. Try the gentle exercise arts of Tai Chi and QiGong or experience Reiki, Healing Touch or Acupuncture. Look into nutrition and healthy eating options as well as herbal medicine. Holistic healing practices are complementary to your traditional medical needs, therapy and medication.

"Want to pursue a career in healing? There are a variety of certification courses and training available. During my studies at the Barbara Brennan School of Healing back in 1990, students from California were doing Reiki and I became a Reiki Practitioner and then a Reiki Master so I could teach this gentle effective energy modality. As the population around the world continues to age, caring compassionate services and the healing professions will be in high demand despite the advent of AI (Artificial Intelligence). Humanity will need assistance adjusting to the rapid earth changes as life continues to move at a faster and faster pace."

Elsie's Tips:

- One-Minute Meditation ~ Place one hand over the other at the heart energy center right between the breasts. Take a deep breath. Now, breathe in peace, calm and resilience; breathe out stress and anxiety. Just let go. Do this slowly for three breaths or more if needed.

- Calm & Restore ~ Place your fingertips on each side of the right and left temples. Take a breath in and smooth over the ears to the end of the earlobe. Go back to the temples and repeat 4 to 5 times. On the last soothing sweep, land on your heart energy center between the breasts and take a body check.

- Caution! That voice of inner judgment, the great saboteur will jump into action and try and tell you this won't work for you but everyone else. Or, you can't hold yourself in love; or, don't make changes, stay in the old familiar living mode.

- Action! Fire that voice of inner judgment. Don't buy into that criticism, doubt and fear. You have an innate inner intelligence that keeps you breathing, walking and talking every moment of the day. Your body, mind and spirit has enormous healing capacity. Take time every day to tap into this reservoir of unlimited potential! Create a partnership with this healing wisdom for health, vitality and resilience!

Here is a quote from me with love and light.

"Hold all of your being in love, honor and reverence just as you are in the moment!"

~Elsie

REAL LIFE HERO TODD FORTIN - COMPUTER ENGINEER

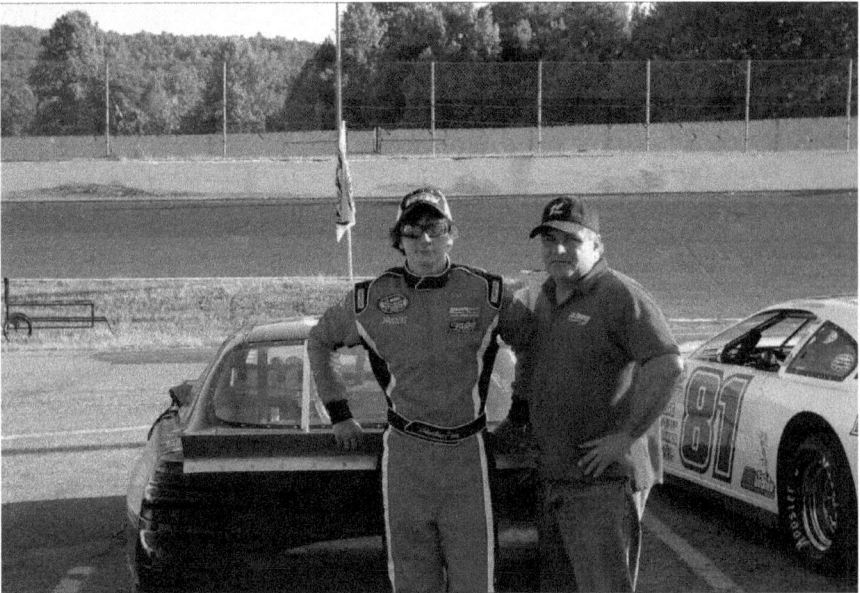

Left: Jonathan Fortin; Right: Todd Fortin

A single parent with, military-style character, allowed no one to interfere while focusing on the most important aspect of his life, his son. The world of car racing was exciting, costly and required hard training. A strict responsibility was a must, maintaining a balance between school and racing and it was his job as a parent to make that happen. Studies could not and would not suffer. A father, a teacher, a protector, and a guide in life.

A real life hero. A serviceman that we thank for our freedom. A parent that knew his job, he created and supported opportunity for his child, all the while teaching and guiding his son on how to maneuver life and make split-second decisions. He understood that we teach our children right from wrong building a strong foundation, showing them the way to maintaining finances and health, and protecting themselves from the negative forces in life. Todd stays close to his son, his best friend, life's greatest endeavor.

"I was 24 years old living the life of a superstar, a college graduate and a job to die for. With plenty of cash to spare, driving a Porsche and a house in Cocoa Beach, Fl, suddenly the hammer was lowered, I lost my job. With no more money coming in, it was imperative that I put a plan in place fast! The military had a hiring freeze on, so I enlisted in the Navy, for 12 years and obtained an Oceanographic degree. Working as a sonar technician in the 'cold war,' tracking the Soviet submarine Oscar in deep waters, brought an accommodation award and shore duty of my choice for the next four years in Mayport, Florida. After flight training and opening a Dive Shop, I found myself in a divorce with full custody of my five-month-old son. So my fatherly responsibilities began: parent, disciplinarian, financial expert, head of household and provider. A new challenge was at hand and I accepted it with honor."

Military Service Pros:

- Rise above others due to the competitive nature of the Navy
- Education paid and degrees obtained
- Pension
- Healthcare

Military Service Cons:

- Away for long periods
- Hardship when re-entering into society
- Status changes from service life to civilian life

Todd's Tips:

- Live life your way.
- Recommends military service life to obtain education.
- Join ROTC in High School.
- Be financially stable, have a strong foundation in place, and be responsible before becoming a parent.
- Be ready mentally to take care of another human being.
- The Service will change you into a responsible, honorable adult.
- Do it right the first time.

REAL LIFE HERO JULIE REARDON - REGISTERED NURSE AND REALTOR

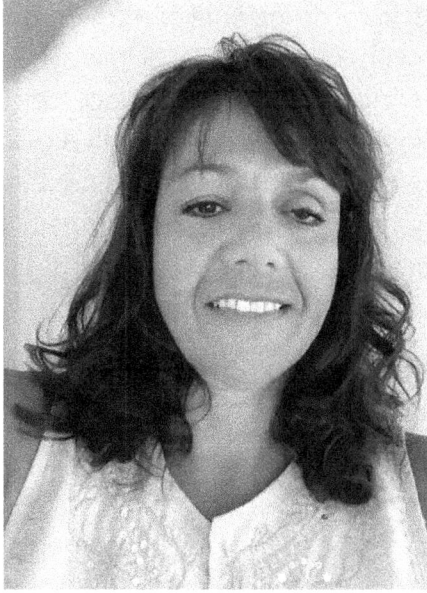

Strong, competent, intelligent, compassionate and kind are just a few qualities that Julie beholds. Decision-making comes with ease and her take-charge manner keeps the team strong and flowing without disruption. When there is a stance to be taken, there is no second guessing and the right path will always be chosen. It is a blessing to have a such a friend at your side, she will always have your back.

A leader and hero. A career and businesswoman. Julie is a picture of strength and integrity. Intelligent and beautiful with a quick wit, taking on responsibility comes second nature. Always taking the path least traveled, Julie does the right thing and makes the right choices. A friend forever, she is more like a sister. As you go through life there are some that you will never forget and she is one of them.

"My name is Julie. I have been a registered nurse for almost twenty years. This is the second career of three.

For as long as I can remember I have always wanted to be a nurse. However, with less than stellar grades in chemistry and advanced math classes in high school and fear of failure created in my mind, I chose an alternative path. Strong urging from my mother spearheaded a business education upon graduating from high school. I graduated from a business school and spent fifteen years in the business field with positions ranging from an executive assistant to an outside sales representative.

Upon getting married and greatly dissatisfied with my business career despite my successes, I decided to revisit the pursuit of my the lifelong goal of becoming a nurse. Having to help support a mortgage, car payments, and living expenses, I was not fortunate enough to just be a student and had to create a transition plan. I started by taking the core classes of anatomy, physiology and chemistry, apprehensively, of course, based on my past performances. I took one class at a time. Additionally, I took a course and became an Emergency Medical Technician in an effort to gain experience and keep up with my living expenses. Fortunately, this certification allowed me to obtain a job in a busy Emergency Department that satisfied both of my objectives. Then, I went through a divorce. This is where perseverance pays off. I had to move, continue working full time, going to college full time and juggle an ever-changing schedule. Consequently, I had to take on a waitressing job in addition to a full load of responsibilities to reach my goal. In 2001, I graduated from nursing school and started my lifelong dream. Now, no career is perfect and with everything in life, we fall down but have to get up. These days I go home and feel that I really helped someone or made their quality of life better based on their expressed gratitude, which is all the gratification I need for the sacrifices I made to feel successful.

"After becoming satisfied with my success in nursing, I decided it was time to create new goals. It would have to be a hobby, though. I still had life's financial responsibilities and would not be able to leave my job. I had always had an interest in remodeling houses and had dabbled in it to this point but had owned and lived in them at the same time. I wanted a project that was independent from my current home. I had tried to fulfill this need years ago but had failed because I did not have the financial component secured and abandoned the idea at that time. Now, some 10 years later, I was ready to try again.

"At the suggestion of a friend, I went to a local bank that specialized in commercial loans. Once I was advised of the working capital that I needed to accomplish this, I figured out a way to procure it. Then, I had to visit many vendors and suppliers to figure out how I could accomplish the remodel with this minimal budget. Although the budget for the first house was very small, I purchased the home, remodeled it, and sold it within eight months. Now this may not seem like any great feat to some of you but as a single woman without any construction training or experience, it was the stepping stone for my future remodels."

Julie's Tips:
- Start with a plan.
- We all have to start somewhere, but it's not where you start, it's where you finish.
- The hardest part of getting what you want is knowing what you want. The easy part is figuring out a way to get it. Good Luck!!!

REAL LIFE HERO DEBRAH URBANSKI - REGISTERED NURSE AND SERVICE MOM

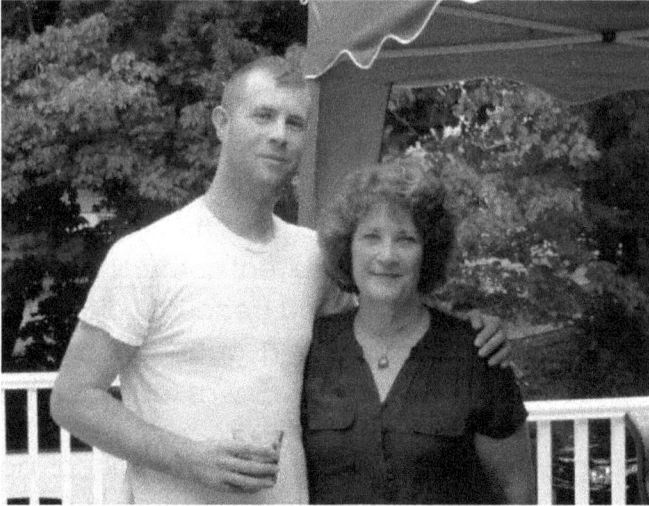

A kind soul and a superb nurse. What you say matters. Genuine, loving, caring and a friend forever. It was an honor to work side by side with such a highly regarded individual. She is in a class all of her own.

A hero's hero. A serviceman's mom, we thank both Deb and her son for our freedom. Deb's maturity, understanding, faith and support allowed her son to leave for the service and return home. The fight is real. A woman of strength, compassion and faith helped her through trying times when her son was away and then upon returning. She was living what some only hear about. Her son had to reintegrate into society as a civilian and our servicemen and women are at the highest risk for Post Traumatic Distress Syndrome (PTSD). Her love and strength are unbreakable. Fearful that your child may not make it home, or wondering how fragile the human mind may become with the visions of service, yet so proud of the man or woman they have become. The bond of a mother and son is unbreakable, just like their faith.

"Our son Ryan came home one day and announced that he had been meeting with a recruiter. He had decided to join the army. I was of course alarmed. We were at war.

"He had since a young age had an interest in military play. Camouflage and weapons. But it still took me by surprise. Ryan already finished college receiving a degree in Criminal Justice. But getting a job in law enforcement seemed impossible. He started working with his dad in HVAC. I knew he was having trouble finding his way. I prayed and prayed for God to help him find his way. But joining the army? That is not the answer I expected, dear Lord. God hears us and the answers are sometimes very unexpected. Ryan signed October 2011. Five years active, three years inactive.

"My husband and I had no experience with the military. Our dads were in the Navy during WW2, that was it. There is a lot to learn. The military has its own language. We were given pamphlets of info to explain how the army works. It was important to figure out what the abbreviations meant. For instance, Ryan's job, MOS, was military police, MP.

"Out of basic, he was immediately sent to Korea for one year. When he was able to call or Skype home, it was for a limited time with sometimes faulty connections. Conversation was easier if we understood most of his verbiage and he didn't have to explain what he was talking about.

"I was his emergency contact. I learned quickly never turn off my cell phone. Even at work. He learned quickly that he should have notified his bank and credit card company he was going to Korea. His accounts were shut off. For security of course. Also, his cell phone. While out of the country he couldn't use Sprint. He had to sign up with another provider. In order to put his Sprint account on hold and reactivate his bank accounts, it was necessary for me to make lots of phone calls. FAX my POA status documents to the proper places. Ryan couldn't do it from Korea. It would've been less stressful had we known to do this ahead of time. After serving one year in Korea, he was sent to Lewis McChord in Washington State for the next four years.

"While Ryan was in the army, my husband and I lost our dads. My husband's dad in 2012 and mine in 2013. We have small families and Ryan was close to both of his grandfathers. It was shocking to us that a grandfather is not considered an immediate family member. Therefore it is up to the discretion of his commander whether he could get granted leave to come home for the funeral. I was to call the Red Cross. A very nice man asked me specific questions about the relationship Ryan had with his grandfather. I answered truthfully. No, he never lived with him. No, he was not financially supported by his grandfather. The Red Cross then contacts the commander to request the soldiers leave. My dad had just died. It was inconceivable to me that Ryan may not be allowed to come home. I needed him here. He needed to be here. I felt so distraught, so out of control. In the end, he was allowed leave for both funerals. In the case of my own father, he had taken ill suddenly. He died two weeks before Christmas. This allowed Ryan to be home for the holidays. My prayers included thanking God for this timing. I knew Ryan was homesick and I missed him so much. Him being home with family did us all wonders. It was a bittersweet time for sure.

"Ryan's time in the army was, of course, full of ups and downs. He was homesick for sure. I tried to include him on social media during family gatherings. During phone calls, he didn't always want to talk about what was happening in his life out there. He wanted to hear about home life. His cat. Or what we were having for dinner. Or Boston happenings, especially sports. I sent packages of baked goods. He treasured his Boston Strong t-shirt and cup. I was dying to hear about his day, his life, but didn't press it. I had to let the brief time on the phone or Skype be his.

"I do remember a couple phone calls when he said he wasn't going to make it. He had to get out. He was never specific about any problem, just so very sad.

"I realized there's not much I can do to help him. Who do you call? I prayed. Please give him strength. I tried to say not much longer, but that wasn't true. I tried to say, at least you're not in the Middle East, but that made him feel worse I think. I asked him to see someone to talk to. But there was, in the end, nothing I could do. Helpless, without any control of the situation.

"He was in. He signed the papers. It was all on him, sink or swim. It was only after he was discharged and home that he started talking about it.

"His dark times. Washington is rainy and grey. You rarely see the sun. During his time there, we had a government shutdown. His pay was briefly in jeopardy. The government was cutting the military budget. Little to no promotions were being given which meant no raise in pay. I learned that governments matter. What the president says and does matter. I shouldn't say anymore about that.

"He was working 12-hour shifts, days on end. Morale was way down on the base. Which meant many calls for domestic violence and suicides. The base is like a huge city. Being an MP on the road, he was often first on the scene. Dangerous and gruesome at times. His memories turn to nightmares still.

"I can not speak to how he got through it all. I know he did not seek counseling. Stigma maybe? Ryan gives us the credit. His solid upbringing. Our strong work ethics. I do believe though that his fellow soldiers got him through it. They get each other through the tough times. One of his best army buddies was here on a visit once. He told me they would go to Ryan's barracks and make him come out with them. I believe It is true that no one can understand unless you've been there. These are friends he will have for life.

"It was certainly not all bad times. He has happy memories and lots of great stories. We were very blessed that we had the means to visit Washington three years in a row. We went at Thanksgiving time, renting a house. We were able to host his soldier friends. Hear the banter. See the camaraderie between them. Watch them eat a home-cooked meal. Be part of his life.

"Ryan received many accommodations while in the army. Two army achievement medals. An army commendation medal. And a very difficult to get Good Conduct award. He was team leader for his years in Washington, being responsible for soldiers 24/7 who were assigned to him. In Korea, he was he did private security detail for a 4-star general.

"For one more year, Ryan is on inactive duty. He has declined any offers to re-sign. I told him he has served his country proudly. In two weeks he will graduate from the Police Academy. Army Specialist will soon be Officer.

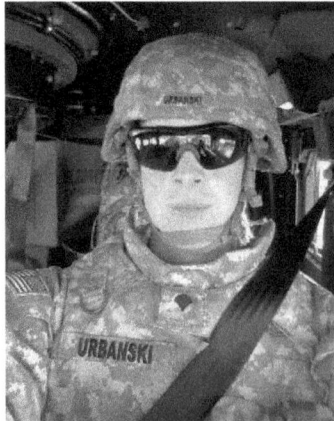

"His civilian life is taking shape. Now my prayers are of thanks and will be for his safety as a police officer. Takes a special person to live the life he is living. I am so proud of his strength."

Deb's Tips: (To the parent of a child who wants to join the military)
"Keep calm and be positive. Although it is not for everyone, most who join have lasting memories and friendships. Pride in succeeding gives lifelong confidence.

"In hindsight, I would advise my son to save money as best you can while in. The paychecks in the Army were small but so were the daily living expenses. These guys work hard and love their free time, partying costs a lot. Use your education benefits and take a class. Once out, the cost of living is a shock!

"Our son, thankfully, was wise when he went in. He saw many a soldier though make the mistake of getting married while enlisted. It sounds crazy but I heard many stories from him about this and it's a thing.

"There are actually women out there who want the benefits offered by the government. Health insurance, cheap housing, etc. The bars and clubs near the base are targeted by these women. Marrying a soldier they know there is a good chance the soldier will be deployed for periods of time.

"Ryan saw many a miserable soldier, some as young as 19, having marital problems. My opinion; the soldier joins, leaves home young, with no life experience and get lonely. They call these women 'dependopotomus'.

"Another reason some soldiers marry is thought out and planned. The soldier can get on-base housing when married. Definitely a step-up from living in a barracks. Neither of these scenarios is something we experienced, just hearsay.

"Be the one phone call that he can make to hear about home. Don't push to hear about his life. His life is mostly difficult, hard. He gets through it in his own way. But when he calls, let him direct the conversation. If he wants to tell you about his day fine. But he may want to hear about home, or his cat. It's hard for the parents when he's far away. You feel guilty. You don't want to tell about family gatherings and things he has missed, but you can and should. He wants to be a part of it, to know what's going on. The soldier needs this connection to his family."

INDUSTRY LEADERS AND THE PAVED PATH

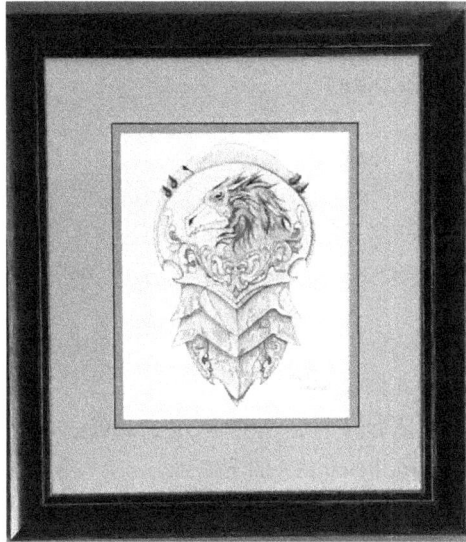

Artist Alisa Chmielinski

You will hear a lot about success throughout your lifetime and you will be the decision maker in what that definition means. Whether you're a seven-figure speaker, someone who has broken free from a bad environment and striving to live a peaceful life, or maintaining a healthy family lifestyle, it all comes down to what you believe in and strive for.

Sometimes, along the way, you may need guidance, direction, or just a lending ear to talk through the plan. The bottom line secret is, you are worth it and no one can take away your hopes, dreams, and spirit.

It can all start with a plan and focus, focus on the greater good. Often the question is "Where do I start or who do I believe?" The beginning is understanding, and until you have decided what will make you happy, please let some industry leaders teach you what they have been through, and how they have tried to make your future path to success easier, by way of words.

Build that foundation of knowledge, belong to something you like to do, or find relaxing.

How about a good read?

Industry leaders have paved a path of success, I show you a personal library of good reading. See below:

1. Bolt, Chandler. (2016) Published. CreateSpace Independent Publishing Platform.
2. West, Kay. (2001) How To Raise a Gentleman. Nashville, Tennessee: Rutledge Hill Press.
3. Bridges, John and Curtis. (2001) As A Gentleman Would Say.Nashville, Tennessee: Rutledge Hill Press.
4. West, Kay. (2001) How To Raise A Lady.Nashville, Tennessee: Thomas Nelson.
5. Shade, Sheryl. (2004) As A lady Would Say. Rutledge Hill Press
6. Brunson, Russell. (2017) The Funnel Hacker's Cookbook. ClickFunnels
7. Steinberg, Michael. (2000) New York Institute of Finance Guide to Investing. Prentice Hall Press.
8. Morrison, Anthony. (2008) The Hidden Millionaire. Morrison Publishing.
9. Morrison, Anthony. (2011) Advertising Profits From Home. Visionary Strategies.

10. Morris, Tom. (1998) If Aristotle Ran General Motors. Holt Paperbacks.
11. Stanley, Thomas J. (2010) The Millionaire Mind. Rosetta Books.
12. Kaufman, Josh. (2013) The First 20 Hours. Portfolio.
13. Loehr, Jim and artz, Tony. (2003) The Power of Full Engagement. Free Press.
14. Cabane, Olivia Fox. (2012) The Charisma Myth. Portfolio.
15. Vaynerchuk, Gary. (2009) Why Now Is The Time To Crush It. Harper Collins Publisher
16. Sanborn, Mark. (2006) You Don't Need A Title To Be A Leader. Currency.
17. Bradberry, Travis and Greaves, Jean. (2009) Emotional Intelligence 2.0. TalentSmart.
18. Mandino, OG. (2011) The Greatest Salesman in the World. Bantam.
19. Maxwell, John C. (2007) The 21 Indispensable Qualities Of A Leader. Harper Collins Leadership.
20. Ehrenreich, Barbara. (2010) Nickel and Dimed. Metropolitan Books.
21. Macleod, Hugh. (2009) Ignore Everybody. Portfolio.
22. Sasevich, Lisa. (2015)The Live Sassy Formula. Sassy Press.
23. Turner, Josh. (2017) Booked. Josh Turner.
24. Weathington, Richard and Ley, Beth M. (2007) Mortgage-Free For Life. BL Publications.
25. Kennedy, Dan. (2004) No B.S. Business Success. Entrepreneur Press.
26. Covey, Stephen. (2017) The 7 Habits Of Highly Effective People. Mango.
27. Harvard Business Review. (2011) Collaborating Effectively. Harvard Business Review Press.
28. Trump, Donald J., and Zanker, Bill. (2007) Think Big And Kick Ass. Harpers.

29. Carnegie, Dale. (1998) How To Win Friends & Influence People. Pocketbooks.
30. Lechter, Sharon L., and Reid, Greg S. (2011) Three Feet from Gold. Sterling.
31. Singer, Blair. (2012) Sales Dogs. RDA Press, LLC.
32. Rohn, Jim. (1991) The Five Major Pieces to the Life Puzzle. Jim Rohn International.
33. Rohn, Jim. (1981) The Seasons Of Life. Jim Rohn International.
34. Miller, Brian Cole. (2015) Quick Team-Building Activities for Busy Managers. AMACOM.
35. Kiyosaki, Robert T. (2012) The Business Of The 21ST Century. Manjul Publishing House Pvt Ltd.
36. Kiyosaki, Robert T., and Lechter, Sharon. (2008) The Business School. KW Publishers Pvt Ltd.
37. Failla, Don. (2010) The 45-Second Presentation That Will Change Your Life. Sound Concepts, INC.
38. Kiyosaki, Robert T., and Lechter, Sharon L. (2011) Cashflow Quadrant. Plata Publishing.
39. Allen, Robert G. (2008) Multiple Streams Of Income. Wiley.
40. Trudeau, Kevin. (2011)Free Money. Vanguard Press.
41. Stanley, Thomas J., and Danko, William. (2010) The Millionaire Next Door. Rosetta Books.
42. Levitt, Arthur. (2003) Take On The Street. Vintage.
43. Singer, Blair. (2013) Little Voice Mastery. XCEL Press.
44. Fenton, Richard, and Waltz, Andrea. (2011) Go For No. Courage Crafters, INC.
45. Buckingham, Marcus, and Clifton, Donald O. (2001) Now, Discover Your Strengths. Gallup Press.
46. Hansen, Mark Victor, and Allen, Robert G. (2009) The One Minute Millionaire. Crown Business.
47. Blanchard, Ken. (2002)Whale Done!. Free Press.

48. Hansen, Mark Victor, and Allen, Robert G. (2005)Cracking The Millionaire Code. Crown Business.
49. Kiyosaki, Robert, and Lechter, Sharon L. (2017) Rich Dad, Poor Dad. Plata Publishing.
50. Brinkman, Rick, and Kirschner, Rick. (2012) Dealing With People You Can't Stand. McGraw-Hill Education.
51. DelVecchio, John, and Jacobs, Tom. (2016) Rule Of 72. Sovereign Society.
52. Gladwell, Malcolm. (2007) Blink. Back Bay Books.
53. Ferris, Tim. (2009) The 4-Hour Workweek. Harmony.
54. Gladwell, Malcolm. (2002)The Tipping Point. Back Bay Books.
55. Maxwell, John C. (2007) The 21 Irrefutable Laws Of Leadership. Harper Collins Leadership.
56. Moskowitz, Joel S. (2009) The 16% Solution. Andrews McMeel Publishing.
57. Kiyosaki, Robert T., and Lechter, Sharon L. (2015) Prophecy. Plata Publishing.
58. Graziosi, Dean, (2009) Be A Real Estate Millionaire. Vanguard Press.
59. Yarnwell, Mark, and Yarnell, Rene Reid. (1998) Your First Year In Network Marketing. Prima Publishing.
60. Allen, Robert G. (2003) Creating Wealth with Real Estate. Robert Allen Institute
61. Orberson, Paul. (2007) Something Good's Gonna Happen. Hi-Hope Publishing Company.
62. Robbins, Tony. (2016) Money Master The Game. Simon and Schuster.
63. Cassie, Alex and Cassie, Michael. (2017) The 2% Rule To Get Debt Free Fast. Page Street Publishing.
64. Brunson, Russell. (2017) Expert Secrets. Morgan James Publishing.
65. Pagan, Eben. (2019) Opportunity. Hay House Business.
66. Walker, Jeff. (2014) Launch. Morgan James Publishing.

67. Marshall, Penny. (2013) 80/20 Sales and Marketing. Entrepreneur Press.
68. McElroy, Ken. (2015) The ABC's of Property Management. RDA Press, LLC.
69. McElroy, Ken. (2012) The ABC's of Real Estate Investing.RDA Press, LLC.
70. Sutton, Garrett. (2012) Start Your Own Corporation. RDA Press, LLC.
71. Graziosi, Dean. (2006) Think A Little Different, 4 Volume Set. Think A Little Different.
72. Keller, Gary, and Papasan, Jay. (2012) The One Thing. Austin, Texas: Bard Press.
73. Zarcone, Dana. (2017) Your Shift Matters Breakdown To Breakthrough. DanaZarcone.com
74. Hill, Napoleon. (2016) Think and Grow Rich. Sand Wisdom.

THE CONCLUSION

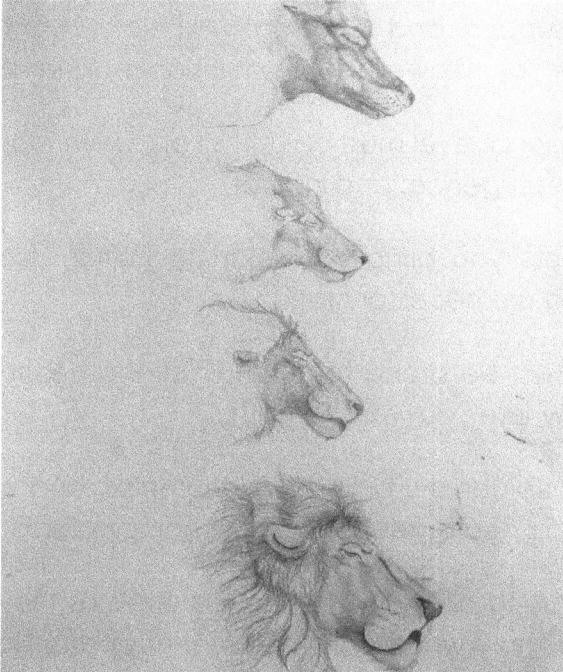

Artist Alisa Chmielinski

As a Warrior faces the future, he first must endure years of training and building what he believes to be his success. With tunnel vision, he cannot be swayed under any circumstance, and his plan is developed with an end goal in mind. He will build upon his strengths which in turn will diminish any weakness. With words unspoken, he proves his almighty strength through action, one of a superior heightened nature. A glance your way will leave an imaginary force that touches only the sense of success. No fool is he for he will prepare that he may lose a battle, but he will win the war.

The path has been paved with clarity, now reach out your hand and take what is yours to be.

The fight has always been for our children, for there is nothing that we will fight harder for than to bring their hopes, dreams, and imaginations to come true. They are our future. Your guidance, support, and teachings will help secure their safety, setting in motion the well-taught decision-making skills.

The foundational level must be unshakable with morals, values, emotional intelligence, and instinct.

Finances help you bring your plan to fruition. Costs will be applied and are necessary to survive.

The body must be strong to maintain strong health and it will get you to where you want to go.

Knowing your identity, building relationships, and maintaining strong mental health keeps your psychological sanity.

Decision-making ability will help avert crises as they arise. You will want to know what to do before it happens. No one goes untouched.

The path has been cleared for you like a road plowed in winter. Take your time, drive carefully, make the right decisions the first time and you will meet success. The Savvy will win the war.

URGENT PLEA

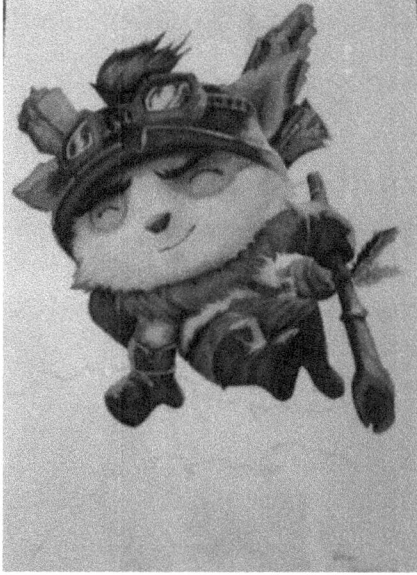

Artist Alisa Chmielinski

THANK YOU FOR READING MY BOOK!

Your thoughts will help make the next version of this book better than ever!

So head on over to Amazon and leave a review, I promise it will not go unnoticed.

Thanks so much!!

~ Robin

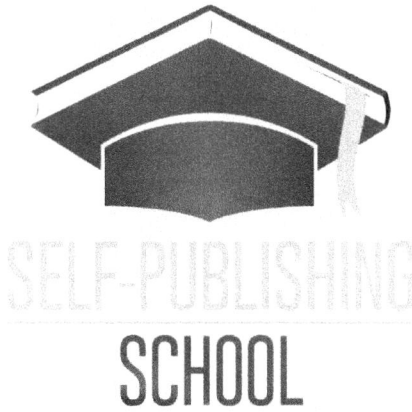

ACKNOWLEDGEMENTS

It is an honor to acknowledge those who understand the importance and live their lives helping others. Your dedication is the future for our children, for without your expertise our children may lose their way. When a child makes a detour it is your strength that will reset the course. You are the glue that holds it all together, you are the superpower, the leaders of life.

A special thank you to the many authors and organizations referenced, for their expertise is second to none.

Our real life Warriors cannot be praised enough, for their stories will live on in the hearts of others. They are fighting life's battles and they are winning.

A special thank you to an elite team of leaders that rise to the present day challenge, striving to extend their hand so they may pull others up to a successful level.

Coach - Marcy Pusey (Self-Publishing School)
Editor - Qat Wanders and Team (Wandering Words Media)
Reference - Wayne Purdin
Formatter - Rachael Cox (Fiverr)
Artist - Alisa Chmielinski
Book Covers - Ida Fia Sveningsson
Book Description - Bryan Cohen (Best Page Forward)
Book Marketing Strategist - Eric V. Van Der Hope

ABOUT THE AUTHOR

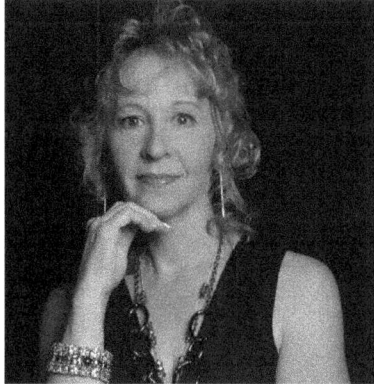

Robin Burnham, first time Author, Mother, and Registered Nurse brings to you, the strength, compassion, and experience needed to empower and raise our youth with warrior expertise and strength. A registered nurse for four decades, split-second decisions became second nature, sometimes it meant saving someone's life. For success starts with the belief of attainment and the tools offered bring the greatest of visions, hopes, and dreams.

Robin was born and raised in Upstate N.Y., a small city named Schenectady. Sch'dy for short, was known as "The Electric City" home of General Electric, it was safe and quiet. It was routine to walk by myself at a young age to elementary school then after school to St. John The Evangelist for catechism, and then home. There were no worries when the kids played all day at Central Park, as long as they were home for dinner. On the weekends, a bike ride to Glenville to play with the cousins was in the plans. You could leave the doors unlocked at night and the windows open without any thought of harm. Carefree, the children played outside all day, climbed trees, played on swings, and played board games. Magical to say the least.

Time is slow when young, wishing you were old enough to drive and get your own apartment. Time is fast when older, almost like a time warp into the future.

When looking back to how things were, to how they are today, one must stop and think of the clear message that has been sent. Our children can only be carefree with the protection of a caretaker at their side.

There is evil lurking and one must ask "Why the change?". Our children must be wise to the world and be alert to the undertow that is playing. The family unit must once again become strong and it is the skill of the caretaker to inform, prepare, and guide. It is our duty to raise our children to be savvy and empower them toward success.

REFERENCES

Chapter 1

[1] Wikipedia. (2018) "The Ethics Centre". Wikipedia Foundation Inc.
https://en.wikipedia.org/wiki/The_Ethics_Centre
[2] The Ethics Centre. "What Is Ethics?". The Ethics Centre.
http://www.ethics.org.au/about/what-is-ethics
[3] Mind Tools Content Team. "What Are Your Values". Mind Tools Ltd, 1996-2019. https://www.mindtools.com/pages/article/newTED_85.htm
[4] Decision-Making-Solutions. "Personal Core Values Help Focus and Align Your Life Choices". Decision Innovation Inc. 2009-2019.
https://www.decision-making-solutions.com/personal_core_values.html
[5] Josephson Institute of Ethics "12 Ethical Principles For Business Executives."
Josephson Institute of Ethics. Used with permission by Michael Josephson,
President & Founder of the Josephson Institute of Ethics.
http://josephsononbusinessethics.com/2010/12/12-ethical-principles-for-business-executives/
[6] Mind Tools Content Team. "Emotional Intelligence in Leadership". Mind
Tools Ltd., 1996-2019.
https://www.mindtools.com/pages/article/newLDR_45.htm
[7] Healthy sense of self. "What Is the Current State of Your Emotional
Intelligence? The Healthy Sense Of Self (2008-2019).
https://healthysenseofself.com/emotional-intelligence/
[8] Bariso, Justin. (2018) "13 Signs Of High Emotional Intelligence". INC.
Manuseto Ventures, 2018. https://www.inc.com/justin-bariso/13-things-emotionally-intelligent-people-do.html
[9] McDermott, David. "Mind control explained - the dangers and how to
protect yourself". Decision-making-confidence 2006-2019.
https://www.decision-making-confidence.com/mind-control.html
[10] Clarke University. (2018) "Tips For Managing Conflict". Clarke University
2006-2019 https://www.clarke.edu/campus-life/health-wellness/counseling/articles-advice/tips-for-managing-conflict/
[11] Bradberry, Travis. (2015) "Are You A Leader Or A Follower?" Talentsmart
Inc. 2019. http://www.talentsmart.com/articles/Are-You-a-Leader-or-a-Follower--2147446613-p-1.html
[12] The Center For Creative Leadership. "The Core Leadership Skills You Need
In Every Role". Center For Creative Leadership 2019. Adapted with
permission from Lead 4 Success: Learn the Essentials of True Leadership,
Center for Creative Leadership, Copyright © 2017.

241

https://www.ccl.org/articles/leading-effectively-articles/fundamental-4-core-leadership-skills-for-every-career-stage/

[13] Milteer, Lee. (2019) Head, Heart and Gut. Albany, New York: Natural Awakenings 2019. https://www.naturalawakeningsmag.com/Inspiration-Archive/Lodestars-of-Powerful-Decision-Making/

[14] Cristen, Rodgers. (2017) "The Difference Between Intuition and Instinct". Exemplore: HubPages Inc. and respective owners 2019. https://exemplore.com/misc/The-Difference-Between-Intuition-and-Instinct

[15] Jacobsen, Annie. (2017) "The US Military Believes People Have A Sixth Sense". Time USA LLC 2019. http://time.com/4721715/phenomena-annie-jacobsen/

[16] EOC Institute "Awakening Intuition: How Meditation Taps The Subconscious Mind". Eoc Institute 2019. https://eocinstitute.org/meditation/how-to-awaken-your-intuition-with-meditation/

[17] Gregoire, Carolyn. "10 Things Highly Intuitive People Do Differently". Huffington Post 2018. https://www.huffingtonpost.ca/entry/the-habits-of-highly-intu_n_4958778

[18] Ishak, Raven. (2017) "11 Ways To Know If Your Intuition Is Trying To Tell You Something & How To Listen". Bustle 2018. https://www.bustle.com/p/11-ways-to-know-if-your-intuition-is-trying-to-tell-you-something-how-to-listen-38787

[19] Ginsberg, Scott. (2014) "The Difference between Instinct and Intuition".Ginsberg, Scott Volume 29: Best of Scott's Blog, Part 15. https://hellomynameisscott.com/the-difference-between-instinct-intution/

[20] Lakhiani, Vishen. "How Intuitive Are You? Take The Quiz and Know Your 6th Sense Score". Finerminds: Mindvalley 2019. https://www.finerminds.com/mind-power/how-intuitive-are-you-quiz/

[21] Schairer, Sara. "What's the Difference Between Empathy, Sympathy, and Compassion?". The Chopra Center at Omni La Costa Resort and Spa 2019. https://chopra.com/articles/whats-the-difference-between-empathy-sympathy-and-compassion

[22] Wikipedia. (2019) "Compassion". Wikipedia 2019. https://en.m.wikipedia.org/wiki/Compassion

[23] Greater Good Magazine. "Empathy Quiz". The Greater Good Science Center at the University of California, Berkeley 2019. https://greatergood.berkeley.edu/quizzes/take_quiz/empathy

[24] Hundt, Isabel. (2016) "Four Signs You May Be An Empath-Warrior". Isabel Hundt 2019. https://www.isabelhundt.com/four-signs-you-may-be-an-empath-warrior/

[25] Orloff, Judith. (2018) "How To Be an Empath Warrior". Psychology Today © 2019 Sussex Publishers LLC. https://www.psychologytoday.com/us/blog/the-empaths-survival-guide/201801/how-be-empath-warrior adapted from https://drjudithorloff.com/empath-survival-guide-description/

[26] Fearless Motivation . (2018) "Stephen Covey Quotes Reveal The Habits Of Highly Effective People". Fearless Motivation Pty LTD. https://www.fearlessmotivation.com/2018/07/31/highly-effective-people-stephen-covey/

[27] Moriarty, Sarah (2016) "Get The 7 Habits of Highly Effective People in 3 Minutes". Blinklist 2019. https://www.blinkist.com/magazine/posts/read-seven-habits-highly-effective-people-3-minutes

Chapter 2

[28] Sadler, Alex Thomas. (2017) "40 Things You Can Do Today To Take Control Of Your Financial Life". Clark Howard Inc. 2019. https://clark.com/personal-finance-credit/easy-ways-to-improve-your-finances-today/

[29] Howard, Clark. (2018) "Free Credit Report Guide". Clark Howard Inc. 2019. https://clark.com/personal-finance-credit/free-credit-report-info/

[30] Hogan, Chris. "How Do I Achieve Financial Freedom". Ramsey Solutions, Lampo Licensing LLC. 2019. https://www.daveramsey.com/blog/what-is-financial-freedom

[31] Thimou, Theo. (2018) "3 Ways To Get A Free VIN Check For Free Before Buying a Used Car". Clark Howard 2019. https://clark.com/cars/free-vin-report/

[32] DaveRamsey.com."Tax Preparation Checklist". Ramsey Solutions, Lampo Licensing LLC. 2019. https://www.daveramsey.com/elp/tax-preparation?&int_cmpgn=no_campaign&int_dept=elp_bu&int_lctn=homepage-smart_moves&int_fmt=text&int_dscpn=Free_Tools_Tax_Checklist_021519#checklist

[33] Wikipedia. (2019) "Fiduciary". Wikipedia Foundation, Inc. 2019. https://en.wikipedia.org/wiki/Fiduciary

[34] U.S. Securities and Exchange Commission (SEC). "Beginners' Guide to Asset Allocation, Diversification, and Rebalancing". Investor.gov. https://www.investor.gov/additional-resources/general-resources/publications-research/info-sheets/beginners%E2%80%99-guide-asset

[35] Town, Phil. "The Rule of 72: "How To Double Your Money Every 7 Years ". Rule 1 Investing 2000-2019. https://www.ruleoneinvesting.com/blog/financial-control/using-the-rule-of-72/

[36] Roth, J.D. (2016) "A brief guide to Financial Freedom". https://www.getrichslowly.org/brief-guide-to-financial-freedom/

[37] BrianTracy.com (Blog) "The 80/20 Rule Explained". Brian Tracy International 2001-2019. https://www.briantracy.com/blog/personal-success/how-to-use-the-80-20-rule-pareto-principle/

[38] Manson, Mark. (2012) "How To 80/20 Your Life". Infinity Squared Media LLC. https://markmanson.net/80-20-your-life

[39] Florida Attorney General. "How to protect yourself: Credit ". State of Florida 2011. http://myfloridalegal.com/pages.nsf/Main/83CAC2FE0EECE15D85257F77004BE173

[40] Sadler, Alex Thomas. (2018) "Free Credit Score Guide". Clark Howard Inc. 2019. https://clark.com/personal-finance-credit/free-credit-score-guide/

[41] DaveRamsey.com "Seven Baby Steps Program". Ramsey Solutions, Lampo Licensing LLC 2019. https://www.daveramsey.com/baby-steps

[42] Adam. (2018) "Buffett's 10/10/10 Rule For Making Financial Decisions". Minafi.com 2016. https://minafi.com/buffetts-10-10-10-rule-for-making-financial-decisions

[43] Tracy, Brian. "7 Point Formula for Financial Freedom, Happiness and Wealth". Brian Tracy International 2001-2019. https://www.briantracy.com/blog/financial-success/7-point-formula-for-financial-freedom-personal-finance-make-more-money/

[44] Better Business Bureau. 10 Steps To Avoid Scams". Council of Better Business Bureaus, Inc. 2019. https://www.bbb.org/avoidscams/

[45] Capital One. (2018) "Protect Yourself Against Credit Card Fraud". Capital One 2019. https://www.capitalone.com/learn-grow/privacy-security/protect-against-credit-card-fraud

[46] USA.gov. (2019) "Report Scams and Frauds". USA.gov. https://www.usa.gov/stop-scams-frauds

[47] Howard, Clark. (2017) "Identity Theft Guide". Clark Howard Inc. 2019. https://clark.com/story/identity-theft-guide/

[48] MoneyTracker.com. "The Budget Kit". Money Tracker 2019. https://www.moneytracker.com/free-printable-budgeting-forms-pdf/

[49] Zdenek, Al. "Are you making the best financial decisions?". Al Zdenek 2019. https://alzdenek.com/assessment-a/

[50] Clearpoint.org. Clearpoint Credit Counseling Solutions, a Division of Money Management International, Inc. https://www.clearpoint.org/resources/ https://www.clearpoint.org/resources/links/

Chapter 3

[51] Stoewen, Debbie L. (2017) "Dimensions of wellness: Change your habits, change your life". National Center for Biotechnology information, U.S National Library of Medicine. https://www.ncbi.nlm.nih.gov/pmc/articles/PMC5508938/

[52] University of Minnesota. "Taking Charge of Your Health & Wellbeing". Regents of the University of Minnesota 2016. https://www.takingcharge.csh.umn.edu/

[53] 16Personalities.com. Neris Analytics Limited 2011-2019. https://www.16personalities.com/free-personality-test https://www.16personalities.com/articles/our-theory

[54] Dodgson, Lindsay. (2018) "What it means to be a type A,B,C, or D personality - and how to find the strength in whatever you are." https://www.msn.com/en-us/lifestyle/smart-living/what-it-means-to-be-a-type-a-b-c-or-d-personality-%E2%80%94-and-how-to-find-the-strength-in-whatever-you-are/ss-BBLF3B4

[55] Psychicguild. "12 Zodiac Signs - Star Sign Dates, Facts and Compatibility". Psychicguild.com 2018. https://www.psychicguild.com/horoscopes_explained.php

[56] Wikipedia. (2019) "Zodiac". Wikimedia Foundation, Inc.
https://en.wikipedia.org/wiki/Zodiac
[57] TakingCharge.csh.umn.edu. Spirituality. Regents of the University of
Minnesota 2016. https://www.takingcharge.csh.umn.edu/what-spirituality
https://www.takingcharge.csh.umn.edu/enhance-your-
wellbeing/purpose/spirituality/why-spirituality-important
https://www.takingcharge.csh.umn.edu/enhance-your-
wellbeing/purpose/spirituality/seven-spiritual-needs
[58] Dienstmann, Giovanni." What is Spirituality-a Guide to Spiritual Disciplines
and Development". Live and dare.com. https://liveanddare.com/what-is-
spirituality/
[59] Kirstie. (2017) "7 Signs you are reaching a higher level of spiritual maturity".
Notmeditating.com. https://www.notmeditating.com/spiritual-maturity/
[60] Robbins, Tony. "Youth Leadership". The Tony Robbins Foundation.
https://www.thetonyrobbinsfoundation.org/
https://www.thetonyrobbinsfoundation.org/programs/youth-leadership/
[61] Katie, Byron. "Do The Work". Byron Katie International, INC.
http://thework.com/en
[62] NeuroNation. "4 Tips for Effective Communication "Neuronation.com.
https://www.neuronation.com/science/tips-effective-communication
[63] Wikipedia. "Albert Mehrabian". Wikimedia Foundation, Inc.
https://en.wikipedia.org/wiki/Albert_Mehrabian
[64] Skillsyouneed.com "Top Tips For Effective Interpersonal Communication"
by Hasib Ahmed. https://www.skillsyouneed.com/rhubarb/effective-
interpersonal-communication.html
[65] West, Kay. (2001) "How to Raise a Lady". Nashville, Tennessee: Rutledge
Hill Press, Nashville, Tennessee. Book.
[66] Mayne, Debbie. (2018) "Social Etiquette Tips". 2018. Dotdash.
https://www.thespruce.com/social-etiquette-tips-1216646
[67] University of Washington. "Healthy vs. Unhealthy Relationships". University
of Washington. http://depts.washington.edu/hhpccweb/health-
resource/healthy-vs-unhealthy-relationships/
[68] Goldsmith Ph.D, Barton. (2011) "10 Truths to Keep Your Relationship
Healthy". Sussex Publishers, LLC., 2019.
https://www.psychologytoday.com/us/blog/emotional-fitness/201107/10-
truths-keep-your-relationship-healthy
[69] Cherry, Kendra. (2019) "Why Parenting Styles Matter When Raising
Children". About, Inc., 2019. https://www.verywellmind.com/parenting-
styles-2795072
[70] Mgbemere, Bianca and Telles, Rachel. (2013) "Types of Parenting Styles
and How To Identify Yours". Developmental Psychology at Vanderbilt.
https://my.vanderbilt.edu/developmentalpsychologyblog/2013/12/types-
of-parenting-styles-and-how-to-identify-yours/
[71] O'Brien, Celeste. (2017) "Parenting Styles and the Highly Sensitive Child".
The AuthenticHSP.com. https://www.theauthentichsp.com/parenting-styles-
highly-sensitive-child/
[72] Johnston, Carly. New England Nutrition Advisors, LLC.
https://nenutritionadvisors.com/

[73] New England Nutrition. (n.d.). Diet and Nutrition Tips.

[74] New England Nutrition. (n.d.). Grocery Shopping Tips.

[75] New England Nutrition. (n.d.). Organic versus NON-ORGANIC

[76] New England Nutrition. (n.d.). HEALTHY FATS.

[77] Kilroy, Dana Sullivan. (2019) Eating the Right Foods for Exercise". Healthline Media, Inc., 2005-2019. https://www.healthline.com/health/fitness-exercise-eating-healthy

[78] Semeco, Arlene. (2018) "Pre-Workout Nutrition: What to Eat Before a Workout". Healthline Media 2005-2019. https://www.healthline.com/nutrition/eat-before-workout

[79] Semeco, Arlene. (2016) "Post-Workout Nutrition: What to Eat After a Workout". Healthline Media 2005-2019. https://www.healthline.com/nutrition/eat-after-workout

[80] PROJECT: PFC brochure. "Our Shakes & Timing". Performance Food Centers, Simple Again, 2019.

[81] Moninger, Jeannette. "8 Diet Rules That Are Meant To Be Broken". Meredith Corporation 2019. https://www.fitnessmagazine.com/weight-loss/eating/8-diet-rules-meant-to-be-broken/

[82] Gunnars, Chris. (2015) "27 Health and Nutrition Tips That Are Actually Evidenced based". Healthline Media 2005-2019. https://www.healthline.com/nutrition/27-health-and-nutrition-tips

[83] Villacorta, Manuel. Huffingtonpost.com "The Best 10 Nutrition Tips From Registered Dietitian Nutritionists". Verizon Media 2019. https://www.huffpost.com/entry/the-best-10-nutrition-tips-from-registered-dietitian-nutritionists_n_9393988

[84] Shapiro, Ira (2018) "Weightlifting is ideal for improving strength, durability and tone at any age". Packet Media LLC, Newspaper Media Group 2019. http://www.centraljersey.com/health/weightlifting-is-ideal-for-improving-strength-durability-and-tone-at/article_acd532e5-ec44-56fa-9fdd-a731ab9f79d1.html

[85] EHStoday. (2009) "Health and Wellness: Exercise Is Important At Any Age". Informa USA, Inc. 2019. https://www.ehstoday.com/health/wellness/exercise-important-all-ages-0309

[86] Wikipedia. "Delayed onset muscle soreness". Wikimedia Foundation, Inc. 2019 https://en.wikipedia.org/wiki/Delayed_onset_muscle_soreness

[87] Fetters, K. Aleisha. (2018) "How to Tell If You Need Electrolytes During Your Workout". U.S. News & World Report L.P.2019 https://health.usnews.com/wellness/fitness/articles/2018-07-13/how-to-tell-if-you-need-electrolytes-during-your-workout

[88] Goldsgym.com/blog "Workout Tips From The Pros". Goldsgym 2019. https://www.goldsgym.com/blog/workout-pro-tips/

[89] Wikipedia. (2019) "Core". Wikimedia Foundation, Inc. https://en.wikipedia.org/wiki/Core_(anatomy)

[90] Go4life.nia.nih.gov "Stay Safe When Exercising In Hot Weather". National Institute on Aging. https://go4life.nia.nih.gov/stay-safe-when-exercising-in-hot-weather/

[91] Go4life.nia.nih.gov "Stay Safe When Exercising In Cold Weather". National Institute on Aging. https://go4life.nia.nih.gov/stay-safe-when-exercising-in-cold-weather/

[92] Go4life.nia.nih.gov "Exercising with Pain". National Institute on Aging. https://go4life.nia.nih.gov/exercising-with-pain/

[93] National Institute of Arthritis and Musculoskeletal and Skin Diseases. "Sports Injuries". National Institutes of Health, U.S. Department of Health and Human Services. https://www.niams.nih.gov/health-topics/sports-injuries

[94] Mike T. "10 Essentials For Survival". Survival Report 2017. https://survivalreport.org/10-essentials-for-survival/

Chapter 4

[95] Mike T. (2017) "7 Basic Human Needs According To Maslow". Survival Report 2018. https://survivalreport.org/basic-human-needs/

[96] Centers for Disease Control and Prevention. "Lightning: Lightning Safety Tips".
U.S. Department of Health & Human Services. USA.gov. https://www.cdc.gov/disasters/lightning/safetytips.html

[97] Weir, Jen. Theoutbound.com "12 Tips For Hiking Safely In Bear Country". The Outbound Collective 2019. https://www.theoutbound.com/jen-weir/12-tips-for-hiking-safely-in-bear-country

[98] USA.gov. "Emergency and Disaster Preparedness". Official Guide to Government Information and Services. https://www.usa.gov/prepare-for-disasters

[99] Godfrey, Lisa J. "A Guide To Adventuring With Your Dog". Adirondack Life Magazine: 2018 Guide To The Great Outdoors. Issue July/August.

[100] Poison Control. "Poison and Prevention". National Capital Poison Center. NCPC 2012-2019. Poison.org https://www.poison.org/

[101] Ready.gov "Snowstorms and Extreme Cold". Department of Homeland Security. https://www.ready.gov/winter-weather

[102] United States Lifesaving Association. "Rip Currents". 6USLA:Association Management Software. This material is the copyrighted property of the United States Lifesaving Association and is used by permission. https://www.usla.org/page/RIPCURRENTS

[103] Office of The Attorney General, Consumer Protection Division. "Hurricane Preparedness Guide". Myfloridalegal.com. http://myfloridalegal.com/webfiles.nsf/WF/JMEE-9KMLPL/$file/HurricanePreparednessGuide.pdf

[104] Ready.gov. "Plan Ahead For Disasters". Department of Homeland Security. https://www.ready.gov/

[105] Thimou, Theo. "29 Items to pack in your emergency kit and bug-out bag". Clark.com; Clark Howard Inc., 2019. https://clark.com/family-lifestyle/29-items-to-pack-in-your-financial-emergency-kit-and-bug-out-bag/

[106] United States Consumer Product Safety Commission. "Protect Your Family From Carbon Monoxide Poisoning". CPSC.gov. https://www.cpsc.gov/safety-education/safety-education-centers/carbon-

monoxide-information-center/protect-your-family-from-carbon-monoxide-poisoning--/

[107] Staysafeonline.org "Digital Declutter". National CyberSecurity Alliance. Stay Safe Online 2019. https://staysafeonline.org/wp-content/uploads/2018/03/DSC-2018-Checklist.pdf

[108] National Highway Traffic Safety Administration. "Winter Driving Tips", "Summer Driving Tips". NHTSA.gov. United States Department of Transportation. https://www.nhtsa.gov/sites/nhtsa.dot.gov/files/documents/14005-winter_driving_tips_2018-2019_110618_v1b_tag.pdf https://www.nhtsa.gov/sites/nhtsa.dot.gov/files/documents/13631-summer_driving_tips_2018_050818_v2_tag.pdf

[109] Mature Driver Course. "Driver & Traffic Knowledge". Driver Educators/Florida Safety Council Chapter 3, 1-11. https://geico.maturedrivertraining.org/

[110] National Institute on Alcohol Abuse and Alcoholism. "Understanding the Dangers of Alcohol Overdose". Pubs.niaaa.nih.gov. USA.gov. https://pubs.niaaa.nih.gov/publications/AlcoholOverdoseFactsheet/Overdosefact.htm

[111] Mothers Against Drunk Driving. "Statistics". MADD.org. MADD 2019. https://www.madd.org/statistics/

[112] The National Domestic Violence Hotline. "What Is Domestic Violence?". The National Domestic Violence Hotline. https://www.thehotline.org/

[113] HelpGuide.org. "Domestic Violence and Abuse". Helpguide.org 1999-2019. https://www.helpguide.org/articles/abuse/domestic-violence-and-abuse.htm/

[114] Hubbard House. "Safety Plan", "Recognize abuse". Hubbard House 2016. https://www.hubbardhouse.org/safety https://www.hubbardhouse.org/thesigns

[115] Brochure. (2018) "High Risk Physical and Behavioral Indicators of Elder Abuse and Neglect". "High Risk Physical and Behavioral Indicators of Domestic Violence". "High Risk Physical and Behavioral Indicators of Child Abuse and Neglect". Received with orientation packet from Old Bridge Medical Center, New Jersey.

[116] Loveisrespect.org. "Boundaries and Expectations". National Domestic Violence Hotline 2017. https://www.loveisrespect.org/content/boundaries-expectations/

[117] RAINN.org "National Sexual Assault Hotline". RAINN 2019. https://www.rainn.org/about-rainn

[118] TraffickingInstitute.org "7 Things Everyone Should Know About Human Trafficking". The Human Trafficking Institute. https://www.traffickinginstitute.org/wp-content/uploads/2017/10/7-things.pdf

[119] Carter, Joe. (2013) "9 Things You Should Know About Human Trafficking". The Gospel Coalition, Inc. 2019. https://www.thegospelcoalition.org/article/9-things-you-should-know-about-human-trafficking/

[120] Polarisproject.org "Recognize The Signs". Polaris 2019.
https://polarisproject.org/human-trafficking/recognize-signs

[121] Office of Juvenile Justice and Delinquency Prevention. "Child Abduction: Resources for Victims and Families". USA.gov.
https://www.ojjdp.gov/childabduction.html

[122] New Jersey Department of Education. "Gang Awareness Guide-Recognize The Signs". New Jersey Office of The Attorney General Juvenile Justice Commission. https://www.nj.gov/lps/gang-signs-bro.pdf

[123] Department of Justice. "Department Of Justice Fact Sheet On MS-13". Justice.gov. https://www.justice.gov/opa/speech/file/958481/download

[124] Kleyman, Katia. ((2018) "18 Terrifying Facts & Stories About MS-13, the World's Most Notorious Gang". Ranker 2019.
https://www.ranker.com/list/mara-salvatrucha-facts-and-stories/katia-kleyman

[125] The Washington Institute. "Ten Things You Need To Know About ISIS". Washingtoninstitute.org. ©2019 The Washington Institute for Near East Policy. Reprinted with permission.
https://www.washingtoninstitute.org/uploads/Documents/infographics/Ten-Things-You-Need-To-Know-About-ISIS_embed.pdf

[126] Jasmine. "What To Do If You Think Your Teen Is Being Recruited by ISIS".
http://time.com/4395269/isis-recruitment-parenting/

[127] Cunningham, David. "Top 5 Questions About the KKK". WGBH Educational Foundation 1996-2019.
http://www.pbs.org/wgbh/americanexperience/features/klansville-faq/

[128] Department of Homeland Security. "Action Guide:Chemical Attacks","Vehicle Ramming", "Fire as a Weapon". DHS.gov.
https://www.dhs.gov/sites/default/files/publications/Chemical%20Attacks%20-%20Security%20Awareness%20for%20ST-CP.PDF
https://www.dhs.gov/sites/default/files/publications/Vehicle%20Ramming%20-%20Security%20Awareness%20for%20ST-CP.PDF
https://www.dhs.gov/sites/default/files/publications/Action-Guide-Fire-as-a-Weapon-11212018-508.pdf

[129] Suicidepreventionlifeline.org "We can all prevent Suicide". The National Prevention Suicide Lifeline. https://suicidepreventionlifeline.org/how-we-can-all-prevent-suicide/

[130] The National Institute of Mental Health. "Suicide in America: Frequently Asked Questions". National Institutes of Health.
https://www.nimh.nih.gov/health/publications/suicide-faq/index.shtml

[131] Stopbullying.gov "What Is Bullying". United States Department of Health and Human Services. https://www.stopbullying.gov/what-is-bullying/index.html

[132] Charactercounts.org "Bullying Matrix", Josephson Institute 2015. Used with permission by Michael Josephson, President & Founder of the Josephson Institute of Ethics. http://charactercounts.org/wp-content/uploads/2014/03/CDS-Bullying-Matrix.pdf

[133] Ren. (2018) "The Opioid Epidemic: How Did We Get Here?". Narconon International. https://www.narconon.org/blog/the-opioid-epidemic-how-did-we-get-here.html?pp=1

[134] Drugabuse.gov "Commonly Abused Drugs". National Institute on Drug Abuse; National Institutes of Health; U.S. Department of Health and Human Services. https://www.drugabuse.gov/drugs-abuse/commonly-abused-drugs-charts

[135] Criminal.findlaw.com "Self-Defense Overview". Thomson Reuters 2019. https://criminal.findlaw.com/criminal-law-basics/self-defense-overview.html

[136] Seltzer Ph.D., Leon. (2015) "Trauma and the Freeze Response: Good, Bad, or Both?". Sussex Publishers, LLC. https://www.psychologytoday.com/us/blog/evolution-the-self/201507/trauma-and-the-freeze-response-good-bad-or-both

[137] Expertsecuritytips.com "The 10 Best Self-Defense Tips for Personal Protection". Expert Security Tips.com 2013-2019. https://www.expertsecuritytips.com/self-defense/

[138] Bishop, Hawk R. "How To Protect Yourself Like A PRO". Hawkbishop.com. http://survivalreport.org/wp-content/uploads/2017/10/How-to-Protect-Yourself-Book-2-2017-.pdf

[139] Reportscam.com. "Top 10- Worst Scams 2018". #Reportscam 2018 https://reportscam.com/worst-scams

[140] USA.gov "Report Scams and Fraud: Most Popular Scams." https://www.usa.gov/stop-scams-frauds

www.ingramcontent.com/pod-product-compliance
Lightning Source LLC
Chambersburg PA
CBHW060314030426
42336CB00011B/1044